Perspective of Recent Advances in Acute Diarrhea

Edited by Sujit K. Bhattacharya

Published in London, United Kingdom

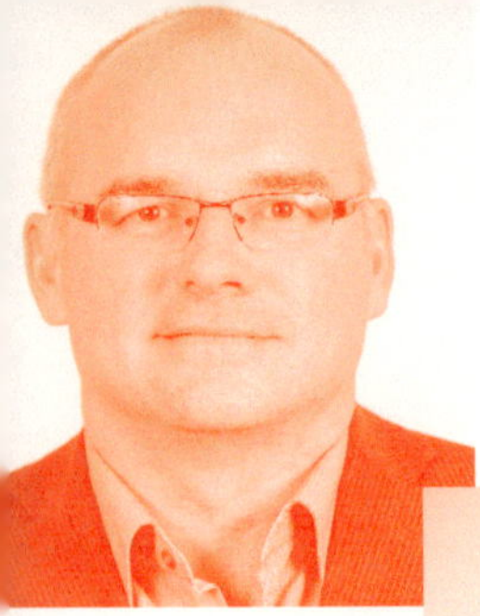
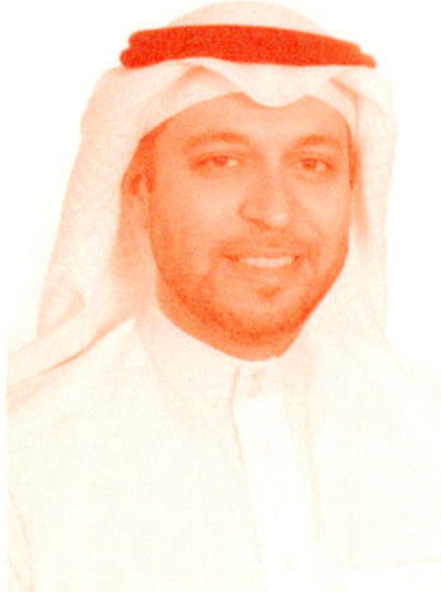
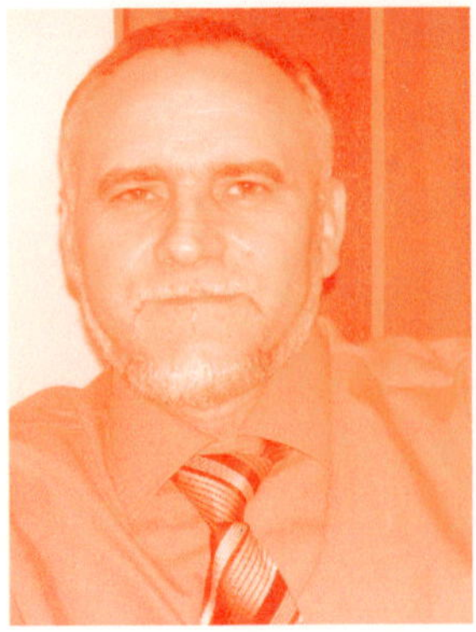
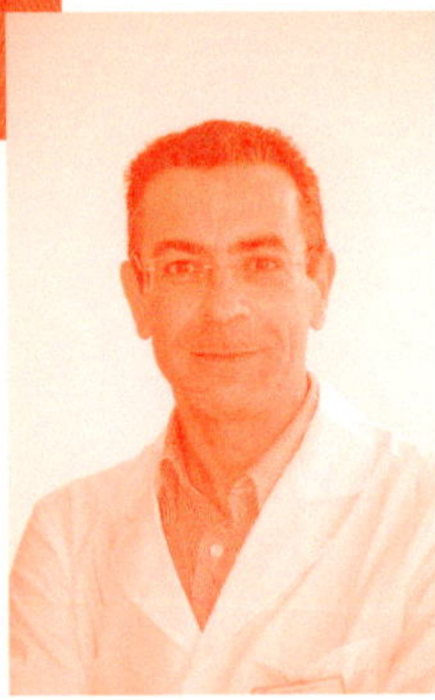
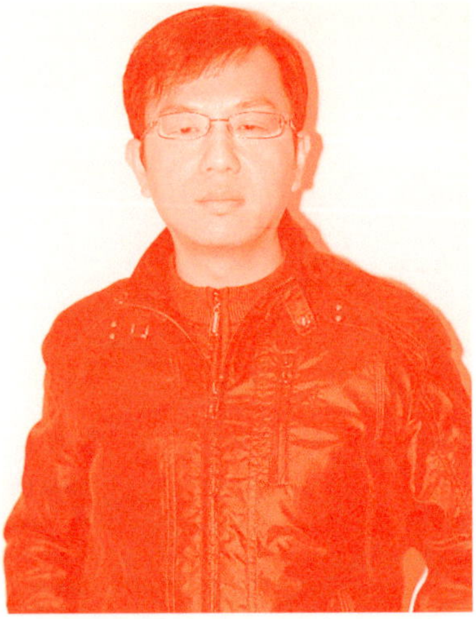
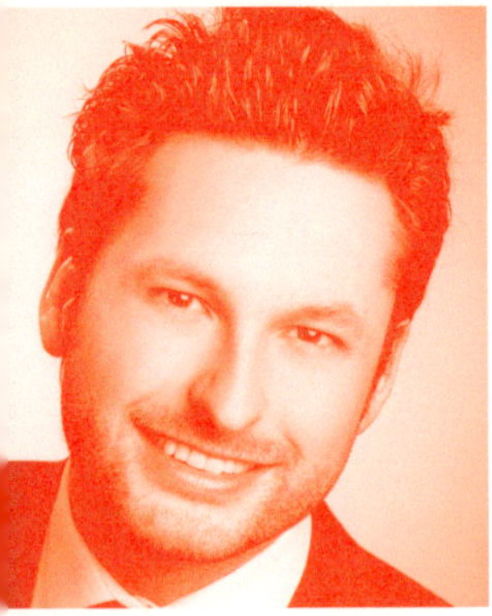
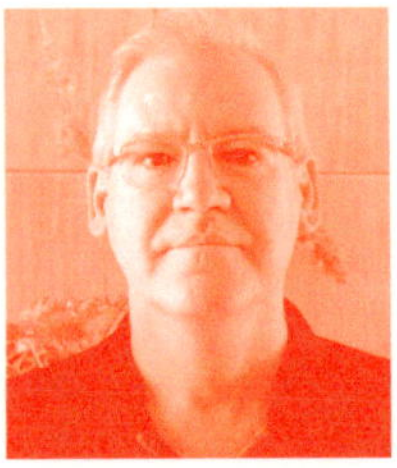

IntechOpen

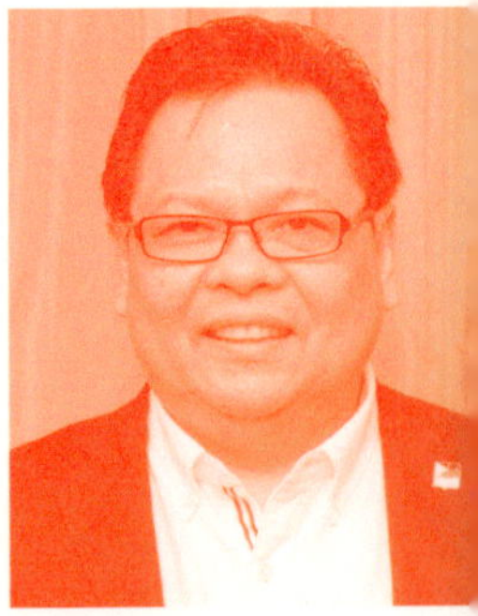
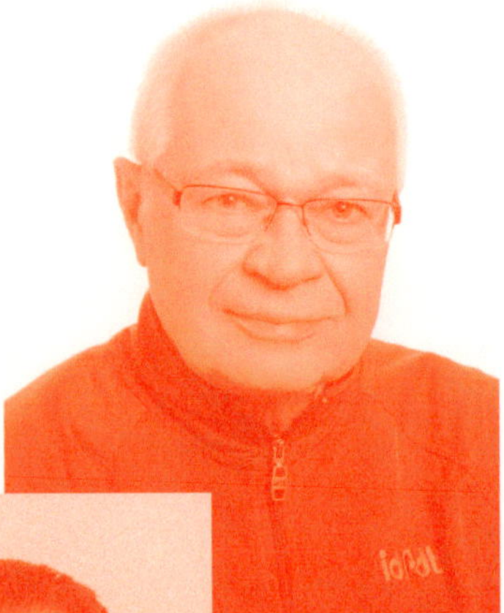
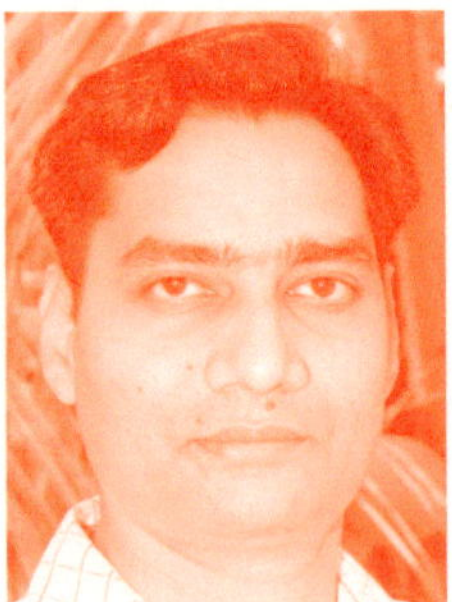
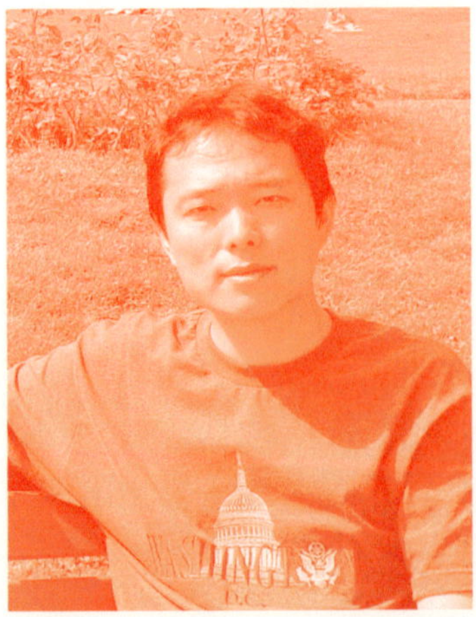
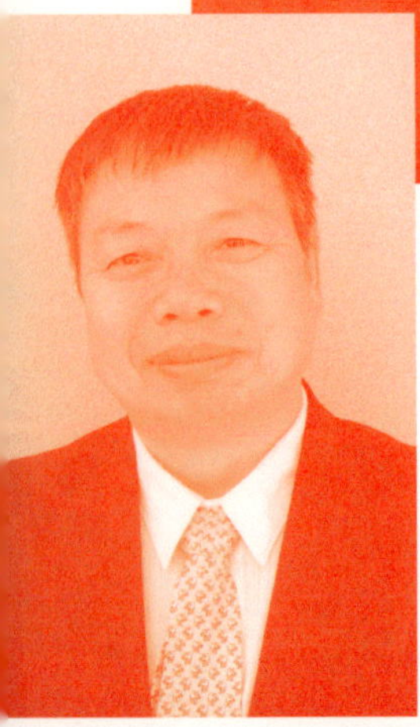
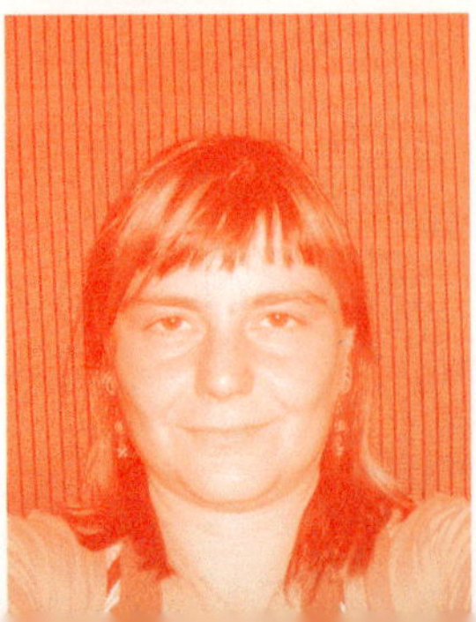

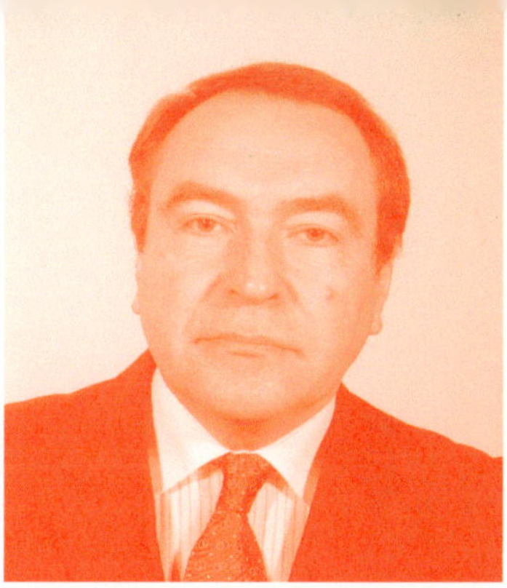

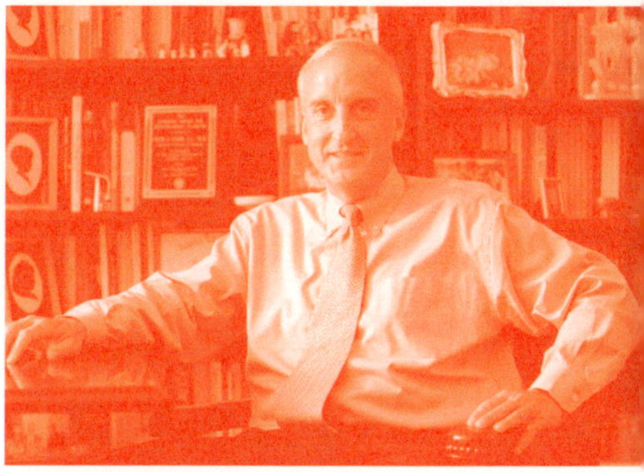

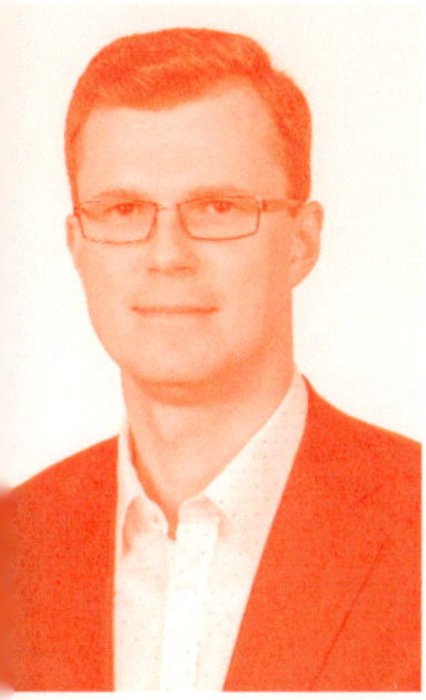

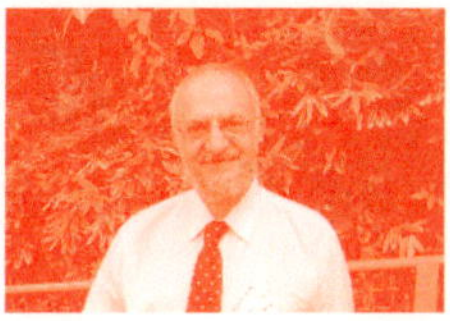

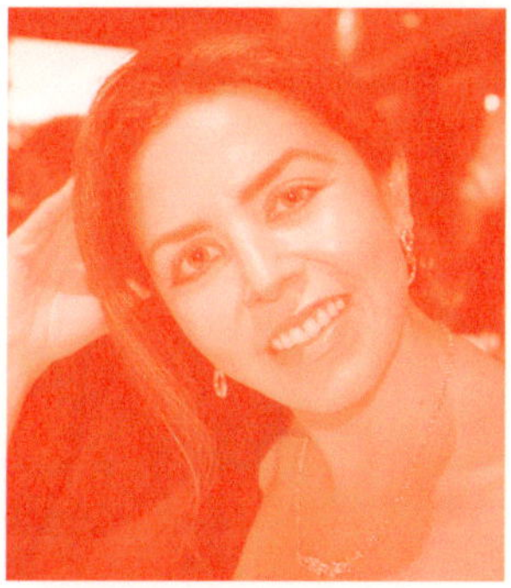

Supporting open minds since 2005

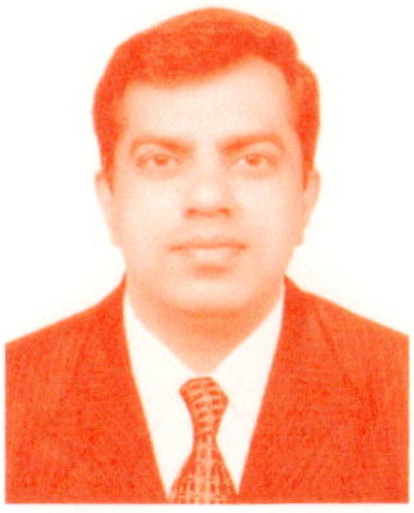

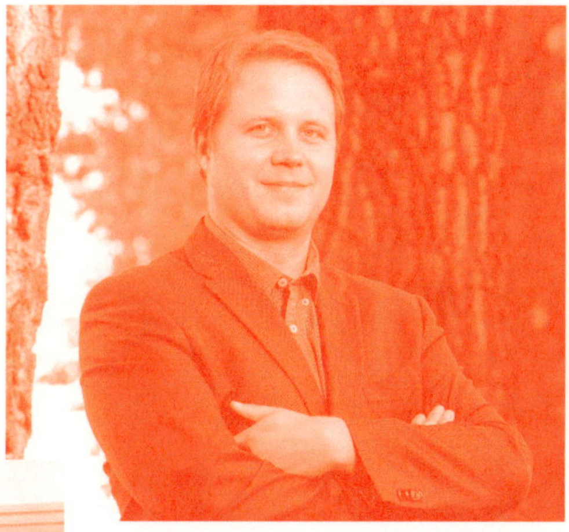

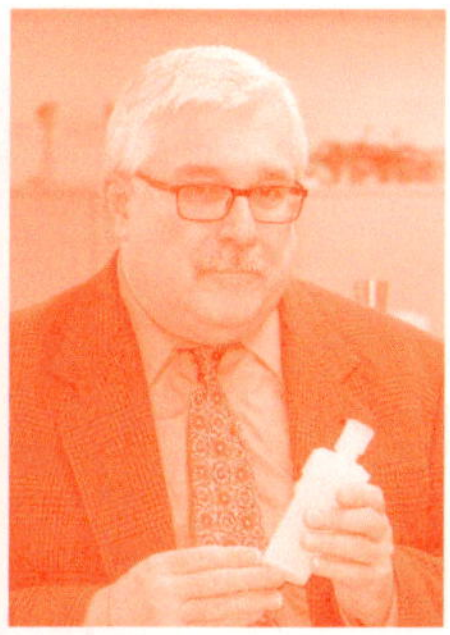

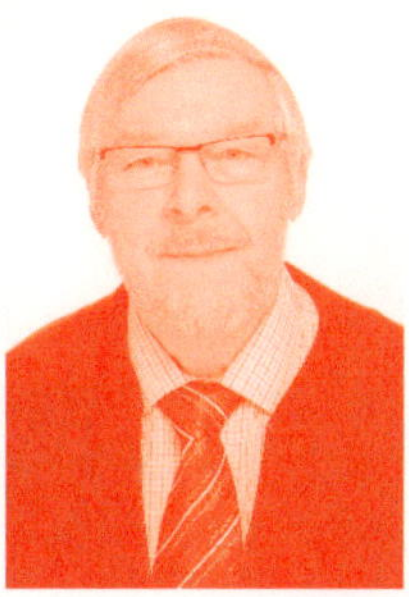

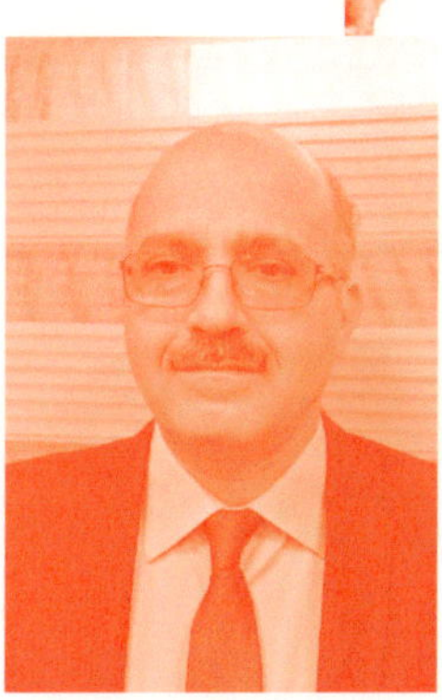

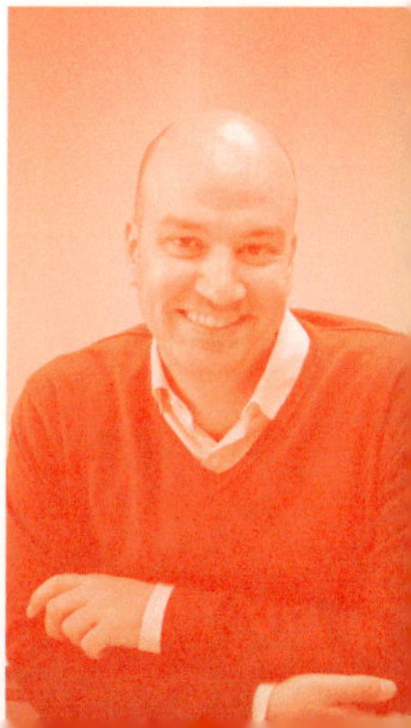

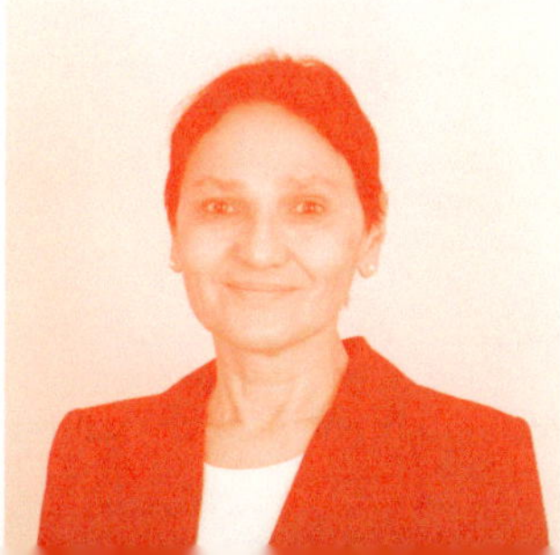

Perspective of Recent Advances in Acute Diarrhea
http://dx.doi.org/10.5772/intechopen.77809
Edited by Sujit K. Bhattacharya

Contributors
Arbianingsih Tiro, Fatihi Hassan Soliman Toaimah, Fysel Manthattil, Muhammad Daniyal, Muhammad Akram, Iftikhar Ahmed Khan, Rida Zainab, Khan Usman Ghani, Masako Kinoshita, Tomohiko Murai, Abhishek Singh, Sujit Bhattacharya

First published in London, United Kingdom, 2020 by IntechOpen
IntechOpen is the global imprint of INTECHOPEN LIMITED, registered in England and Wales, registration number: 11086078, 7th floor, 10 Lower Thames Street, London, EC3R 6AF, United Kingdom
Printed in Croatia

British Library Cataloguing-in-Publication Data
A catalogue record for this book is available from the British Library

Additional hard and PDF copies can be obtained from orders@intechopen.com

Perspective of Recent Advances in Acute Diarrhea
Edited by Sujit K. Bhattacharya
p. cm.
Print ISBN 978-1-78923-865-5
Online ISBN 978-1-78923-866-2
eBook (PDF) ISBN 978-1-78985-356-8

For EU product safety concerns:
IN TECH d.o.o., Prolaz Marije Krucifikse Kozulić 3, 51000 Rijeka, Croatia, info@intechopen.com or visit our website at intechopen.com.

Meet the editor

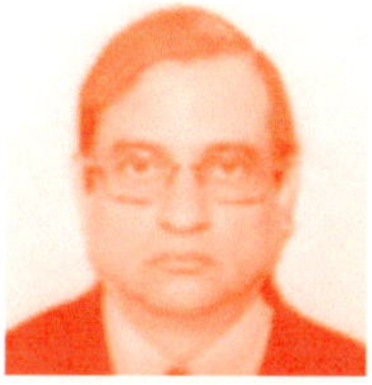

Dr. Sujit K. Bhattacharya obtained his MBBS and MD (General Medicine) degrees from the University of Calcutta. He joined the National Institute of Cholera and Enteric Diseases (NICED), Kolkata, in 1982, and became its Director in 1994. He was appointed Additional Director-General of the Indian Council of Medical Research, New Delhi, in 2006, and joined the World Health Organization in 2009 as a Temporary International Professional. He primarily conducted research on acute diarrheal diseases including cholera, shigellosis, rotavirus, Leishmaniasis, and HIV/AIDS. As a Principal Investigator from NICED, and in collaboration with the International Vaccine Institute, Korea, he conducted the field trial of the oral cholera vaccine in Kolkata along with his team. The vaccine is recommended by WHO for prevention of cholera. He is credited for about 500 publications and has worked in several hospitals in Kolkata during the last five years as Senior Medicine Consultant.

Contents

Preface

Acute diarrhea is mainly a problem in places where sanitation is poor and where there is a lack of clean drinking water and poor personal and domestic hygiene. Acute diarrhea is the second most common cause of childhood mortality. Treatment of acute diarrhea has been simplified with the development of oral rehydration therapy. Rehydration is done on the basis of the degree of dehydration. The current classification of the degree of dehydration has some drawbacks. The new classification method is expected to provide a more simplified method to categorize dehydration. Development of drug resistance among enteric pathogens necessitates the development of safe and effective drugs. Herbal drugs are alternatives. I hope this book will be useful for researchers and clinicians.

I am grateful to the authors who submitted their articles for incorporation in this book. I will be failing if I do not acknowledge the excellent assistance rendered by Ms Kristina Kardum in all stages of preparation of the book.

Sujit K. Bhattacharya
Nirnòy Hospital and Research Centre,
Medinipur, West Bengal, India

Section 1

Introduction

Chapter 1

Introductory Chapter: Perspectives of Recent Advances in Research in Acute Diarrhoeal Diseases

Sujit K. Bhattacharya

1. Introduction

Acute diarrhoea is defined as frequent passage of loose or watery stools mixed with mucus and causes morbidity and mortality particularly in children. The scope of the book is to present information on acute diarrhoeal diseases in relation to clinical features, dehydration, management and prevention. When the stool contains blood, it is called dysentery. Acute diarrhoea is an ancient problem with tremendous public health significance. Acute diarrhoeal diseases comprise of acute watery diarrhoea and acute bloody diarrhoea (dysentery). The prototype of acute watery diarrhoea is cholera, while the same for dysentery is shigellosis. It caused extensive epidemics during flood, famine, war and earthquake when large number of people is shifted to refugee camps.

2. Disease burden

According to an estimate [1] by the World Health Organization, 3–5 million cholera and cholera-like cases occur worldwide, and 100,000–120,000 million cases die with a case-fatality rate of 2.25% (range 1–10%). This figure is actually grossly underestimated, because of under-reporting. These diseases, under the overarching syndrome of acute diarrhoea, cause tremendous pressure on the healthcare delivery system, and during epidemics and pandemics, this is compounded as a real public health problem. There have been seven pandemics (epidemic all over the world) of cholera which spread to more than 102 countries worldwide and killed millions of people.

3. New strain *Vibrio cholerae* O139

An unprecedented happening occurred in the epidemiology of acute diarrhoea [2] when a novel strain of *Vibrio cholerae non* O1 was found to produce an exotoxin akin to cholera toxin and caused large-scale epidemics. The stain was named as *Vibrio cholerae* non O139 Bengal because the strains were isolated from the coastal region of the Bay of Bengal. The disease caused by this stain was indistinguishable from O1 cholera. The same strain of *Vibrio* was isolated from the UK, Germany, the Netherlands, Nepal, Bhutan, Indonesia and Japan. This was thought to be the beginning of eight cholera pandemic, but this actually did not happen so.

4. Etiology

Acute watery diarrhoea comprises of about 20–25 pathogens which fall under the categories of bacterial, viral and parasitic agents. The bacterial pathogens causing diarrhoea include *Vibrio cholerae* O1 and O139, enterotoxigenic *Escherichia coli*, *Vibrio parahaemolyticus* and *Salmonella*; the viral pathogens include *Rotavirus* and *Norwalk virus*; the parasitic agents include *Entamoeba histolytica*, *Giardia lamblia* and *Cryptosporidium*. *Shigella* and *Campylobacter jejuni* cause dysentery. *Rotavirus* is a diarrhoeal disease, which affects children aged between 6 months and 2 years. Early vomiting is an important symptom of *Rotavirus* diarrhoea. Children suffering from *Rotavirus* diarrhoea occupy about 40% of beds in a children hospital.

5. Cholera toxin and dehydration

Vibrio cholerae O1 and O139 produce an exotoxin known as cholera toxin (CT) [2]. CT attaches to gut mucosa and helps in outpouring of fluid and electrolytes, and when the fluid loss exceeds the absorbing capacity of the colon, watery diarrhoea ensues. This leads to a condition called dehydration. Classically, dehydration is categorized as mild, moderate and severe dehydration. Other scoring methods of dehydration have been proposed and will be useful.

6. Management

The treatment of acute diarrhoea is based on the correction of fluid deficit and replacement of ongoing loses. Mild and moderate dehydration can be corrected by oral rehydration therapy [3–6] using oral rehydration salt solution. On the other hand, intravenous fluid is required for the management of severe dehydration. The WHO recommended ORS containing sodium chloride of 2.5 g, potassium chloride of 1.5 g, sodium bicarbonate of 2.9 g and glucose of 20 g dissolved in 1 L of drinking water. ORS is given slowly particularly in children. If vomiting occurs, one has to wait 5–10 minutes and again start giving ORS very slowly. Recently, hypo-osmolar ORS has been recommended. On the clinical aspect of acute diarrhoea, new scoring method has been suggested. It has been reported that epileptic seizures are a manifestation of acute diarrhoea. This is a new area where lots of research may be done.

7. Role of antibiotics

Antibiotics are used in the treatment of acute diarrhoea only for severe cholera and shigellosis. Antibiotic therapy reduces the duration of diarrhoea/dysentery and hastens recovery. The antibiotics of choice for cholera are tetracycline or single dose (300 mg) of doxycycline. Norfloxacin and ciprofloxacin are effective. Herbal medicines may be effective in the treatment of acute diarrhoea. This mode of therapy will be cheap and safe.

8. Drug resistance

Drug-resistant strains of *Vibrio cholerae* have been reported. Shigellosis is treated by various antibiotics including ampicillin, co-trimoxazole, and the fluoroquinolone. However, multiple drug resistance is a huge problem and poses as a therapeutic challenge. The drug resistance is particularly seen in *Shigella dysenteriae* type 1 strains. These strains produced large-scale sporadic, epidemics and pandemic. The drug-resistant shigellosis epidemic that occurred in Bangladesh and Central America caused large morbidity and mortality. A number of complications have been reported in association with *S. dysenteriae* type 1 including hemolytic uremic syndrome (HUS) characterized by hemolysis, renal failure and thrombocytopenia.

9. Prevention

Prevention of acute diarrhoea is a formidable challenge. These include sanitation, safe water and handwashing. Vaccination is an attractive disease prevention strategy. Health education plays a crucial role in the adoption of the strategy, particularly handwashing. This should start at the preschool level to form a habit in later life. Vaccination is an attractive disease prevention strategy. Recently, an oral cholera vaccine has been developed which has been found to protect up to 66% people among those vaccinated [7]. Vaccines against *Rotavirus* are available.

10. Final words

Finally, this book comprises of chapters of topics, which have significance in relation to clinical feature, dehydration, and management and prevention of acute diarrhoea. The reader will find the topics new, informative, and interesting.

Author details

Sujit K. Bhattacharya
Nirnòy Hospital and Research Centre, Medinipur, West Bengal, India

*Address all correspondence to: sujitkbhattacharya@yahoo.com

References

[1] Black RE et al. Global, regional and national causes of child mortality in 2008. A systematic analysis. Lancet. 2010;**375**:1969-1987

[2] Wright EM et al. Coupling between Na+, sugar, and water transport across the intestine. Annals of the New York Academy of Sciences. 2000;**915**:54-66

[3] Bhattacharya SK. History of development of oral rehydration therapy. Indian Journal of Public Health. 1994;**38**(2):39-43

[4] Cholera in Peru. BMJ. 2004;**328**:777

[5] The Lancet Editorial; 1978

[6] WHO. Impact of cholera. 2004 Available from: http://www.who.int/csr/disease/cholera/impactofcholera/en/

[7] Bhattacharya SK et al. 5 year efficacy of bivalent killed whole-cell oral cholera vaccine in Kolkata, India: A cluster-randomized, double-blind, placebo-controlled trial. The Lancet Infectious Diseases. 2013;**13**:1050-1056

Section 2

Childhood Malnutrition

Chapter 2

Childhood Malnutrition in India

Abhishek Singh

Abstract

India is home to 46.6 million stunted children, a third of world's total as per Global Nutrition Report 2018. Nearly half of all under-5 child mortality in India is attributable to undernutrition. Any country cannot aim to attain economic and social development goals without addressing the issue of malnutrition. Poor nutrition in the first 1000 days of a child's life can also lead to stunted growth, which is associated with impaired cognitive ability and reduced school and work performance. Malnutrition in children occurs as a complex interplay among various factors like poverty, maternal health illiteracy, diseases like diarrhoea, home environment, dietary practices, hand washing and other hygiene practices, etc. Low birth weight, episode of diarrhoea within the last 6 months and the presence of developmental delay are often associated with malnutrition in most developing nations including India. This chapter is a small attempt to highlight the state of malnutrition in India and tries to get an insight to overcome the problem. This chapter also highlights the issues and challenges for not obtaining the desired nutritional outcomes. It also provides an insight that this issue can be addressed by adopting comprehensive, coordinated and holistic approach with good governance and help of civil society.

Keywords: childhood malnutrition, determinants, diarrheal diseases, nutritional programmes, challenges

1. Introduction

> *'Good nutrition allows children to survive, grow, develop, learn, play, participate and contribute—while malnutrition robs children of their futures and leaves young lives hanging in the balance'.*

Adequate Nutrition is essential for human development. Malnutrition includes both undernutrition as well as over-nutrition and refers to deficiencies, excesses or imbalances in the intake of energy, protein and/or other nutrients. Benefits of good health are perceived not only at the individual level but also at the level of society and country level as well. Health of an individual is determined by interplay of various factors like social factors, economic factors, dietary factors, lifestyle related factors, environmental factors, government policies and political commitment, etc. [1]. Foundation of an individual's health is laid in early phase of life. It is a well-known fact that in some developing nations, India being one of them, nearly half of children under 5 years of age succumb to death every year due to poor nutrition. It is quite difficult for the poor to bear the cost of treatment especially suddenly occurring out-of-pocket expenditures [2]. A dissimilar trend is observed among individuals of affluent society. Sedentary habits coupled with unhealthy food habits results in weight gain in them. Health experts refer these conditions as malnutrition. The irony is, India being the world's second largest food producer and yet is also home to the large number of undernourished children in the world.

It is well acknowledged that investment in human resource development is a pre requisite for any nation to progress. In year 2012, while releasing HUNGaMA (Hunger and Malnutrition) Report-2011, the then prime minister of India, Dr. Manmohan Singh, expressed dismay at the 'unacceptably high' levels of malnutrition despite high and impressive GDP growth and said it was a matter of 'national shame'. He, being renowned economist, also expressed that that 'the health of our economy and society lies in the health of this generation [3]. We cannot hope for a healthy future for our country with a large number of malnourished children'.

India is home to 46.6 million stunted children, a third of world's total as per Global Nutrition Report 2018. Nearly half of all under-5 child mortality in India is attributable to undernutrition. Children of today are citizens of tomorrow, and hence improving nutritional status of children becomes extremely important. Early childhood constitutes the most crucial period of life, when the foundations are laid for cognitive, social and emotional, language, physical/motor development and cumulative lifelong learning.

Recently Millennium Development Goals (MDGs) has been transformed into Sustainable Developmental Goals (SDGs) and maternal & child health (MCH) has received attention in the last two decades as never before. Adequate nutrition has always been a definitive tool for achieving the maternal and child heath targets. Nutrition is defined as the science of food and its relationship with health. Nutrition is a basic human need and a prerequisite for a healthy life. A proper diet is essential from the very early stages of life for growth, development and for a state of overall well-being. Food consumption, which largely depends on production and distribution, determines nutrition and health of the population. Apart from supplying nutrients, food provides other components (non-nutrient phytochemicals), which have a positive impact on health.

2. Methods for the literature review

We searched PubMed, Google search engine and other databases on the internet for relevant literature. We searched reference lists of all primary and review articles based on the key words 'childhood malnutrition, determinants, diarrheal diseases, India, problem burden, intervention strategies and control program'. Apart from that database of government run nutritional programmes, critical review and analysis of these programmes and related published books were also studied. At few instances, stakeholders of nutritional programmes were also consulted. Relevant data was collected, summarized and analysed.

3. Meaning of malnutrition

Malnutrition is a term that refers to any deficiency, excess or imbalance in somebody's intake of energy and/or nutrients. In simple words, malnutrition can either be due to inadequate intake or an excess intake of calories. The term malnutrition covers two broad groups of conditions namely undernutrition and overnutrition. One is 'undernutrition'—which includes stunting (low height for age), wasting (low weight for height), underweight (low weight for age) and micronutrient deficiencies or insufficiencies (a lack of important vitamins and minerals). Another one is overweight, obesity and diet-related non-communicable diseases (such as heart disease, stroke, diabetes and cancer).

Stunting refers to a child who is too short for his or her age. These children can suffer severe irreversible physical and cognitive damage that accompanies stunted growth. The devastating effects of stunting can last a lifetime and even affect the next generation.

Wasting refers to a child who is too thin for his or her height. Wasting is the result of recent rapid weight loss or the failure to gain weight. A child who is moderately or severely wasted has an increased risk of death, but treatment is possible.

Overweight refers to a child who is too heavy for his or her height. This form of malnutrition results from energy intakes from food and beverages that exceed children's energy requirements. Overweight increases the risk of diet-related non-communicable diseases later in life.

4. Why childhood malnutrition matters to us?

Malnutrition is a universal problem that has many forms. No country is untouched. It affects all geographies, all age groups, rich people and poor people and all sexes. All forms of malnutrition are associated with various forms of ill health and higher levels of mortality. Undernutrition explains around 45% of deaths among children under-5, mainly in low and middle-income countries.

As far as adverse effects of child malnutrition are concerned, growth failure and infections are quite important. Malnourished children do not attain their optimum potential in terms of growth and development, physical capacity to work and economic productivity in later phase of life. It is commonly observed that school absenteeism is much higher in such child that leads to poor performance in the class. Cognitive impairment resulting from malnutrition may result in diminished productivity. Apart from these, Undernutrition increases the risk of infectious diseases like diarrhoea, measles, malaria and pneumonia and chronic malnutrition can impair a young child's physical and mental development. As per estimates of World Bank, childhood stunting may result in a loss of height among adults by 1%, which may further lead to a reduction in individuals economic productivity by 1.4% [4].

Micronutrient deficiencies can lead to poor health and development, particularly in children. Overweight and obesity can lead to diet-related noncommunicable diseases such as heart disease, high blood pressure (hypertension), stroke, diabetes and cancer.

Malnutrition is also a social and economic problem, holding back development across the world with unacceptable human consequences. Malnutrition costs billions of dollars a year and imposes high human capital costs—direct and indirect—on individuals, families and nations. Estimates suggest that malnutrition in all its forms could cost society up to US$3.5 trillion per year, with overweight and obesity alone costing US$500 billion per year [5]. The consequences of malnutrition are increases in childhood death and future adult disability, including diet-related non-communicable diseases (NCDs), as well as enormous economic and human capital costs [6]. According to UNICEF, one in three malnourished children in the world is Indian. It is estimated that reducing malnutrition could add some 3% to India's GDP.

5. The consequences of the problem

- This inter-generational cycle of undernutrition transmitted from mothers to children greatly impacts on India's present and future. Undernourished children are much more likely to suffer from infection and die from common childhood illnesses (diarrhoea, pneumonia, measles, malaria) than well-nourished children.

- According to recent estimates, more than a third of all deaths in children aged 5 years or younger is attributable to undernutrition.

- Undernutrition puts women at a greater risk of pregnancy-related complications and death (obstructed labour and hemorrhage).

- Undernourished boys and girls do not perform as well in school as compared to their well-nourished peers, and as adults they are less productive and make lower wages.

- Widespread child undernutrition greatly impedes India's socio-economic development and potential to reduce poverty [7].

6. Measurement of malnutrition

Underweight is defined as weight that is 2 standard deviations below the WHO child growth standards for that particular age. In other words, child is underweight if Z-scores of child for a given weight for age is less than −2 SD from the median of the WHO/NCHS Child Growth Standards or References.

Wasting is defined as loss of body weight with reference to height. In other words, child is having wasting if Z-scores of child for a given weight for height is less than −2 SD from the median of the WHO/NCHS Child Growth Standards or References.

Wasting is also known as 'acute malnutrition' and is characterized by a rapid deterioration in nutritional status over a short period of time in children under 5 years of age. In children, it can be measured using the weight-for-height nutritional index or mid-upper arm circumference (MUAC). There are different levels of severity of acute malnutrition: moderate acute malnutrition (MAM) and severe acute malnutrition (SAM).

Stunting is defined as a height that is more than 2 standard deviations below the WHO child growth standards median. In other words, child is stunted if Z-scores of child for a given height for age is less than −2 SD from the median of the WHO/NCHS Child Growth Standards or References.

Stunting is also known as 'chronic undernutrition', although this is only one of its causes. Stunting is often associated with cognitive impairments such as delayed motor development, impaired brain function and poor school performance, as it often causes these negative impacts.

7. Magnitude of problem

In present era malnutrition is reflected as double burden, one aspect is undernutrition and other being overnutrition. But, in India and other low and middle-income countries (LMICs), basically malnutrition is synonymous with protein energy malnutrition or undernutrition, which signifies an imbalance between the supply of protein and energy and the body's demand for them to ensure optimal growth and function.

7.1 Global scenario

Globally, approximately 149 million children under-5 suffer from stunting. In 2018, over 49 million children under-5 were wasted and nearly 17 million were severely wasted. There are now over 40 million overweight children globally, an increase of 10 million since 2000 [8]. (**Figures 1–3**) It is estimated that by 2050, 25 million more children than today will be malnourished [9].

7.2 Indian scenario

India is one among the many countries where child undernutrition is severe and also undernutrition is a major underlying cause of child mortality in India. Pattern of stunting prevalence among Indian districts is shown in **Figure 4**.

The prevalence of underweight children under age 5 was an indicator to measure progress towards MDG 1, which aims to halve the proportion of people who suffer from hunger between 1990 and 2015. For India, this would imply a reduction in the child underweight rate from 54.8% in 1990 to 27.4% in 2015. Sustainable development

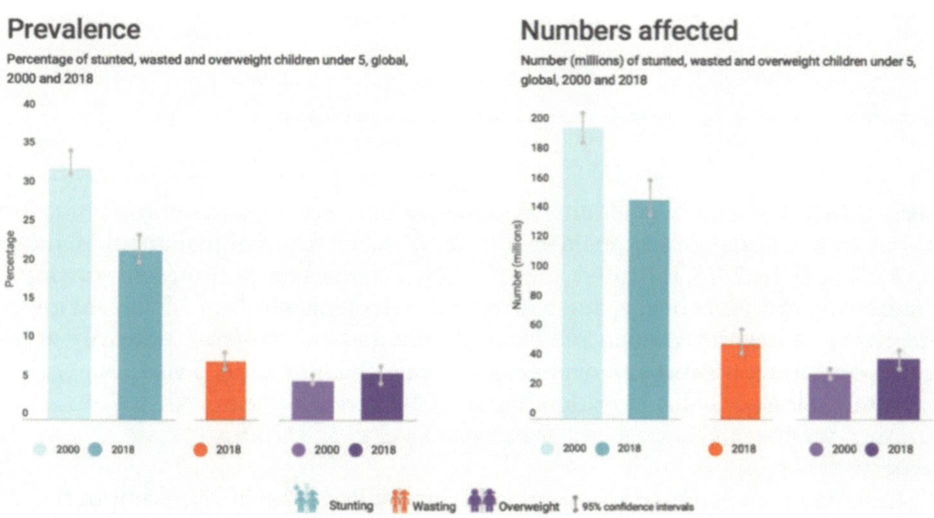

Figure 1.
Global burden of malnourished under-5 children [8].

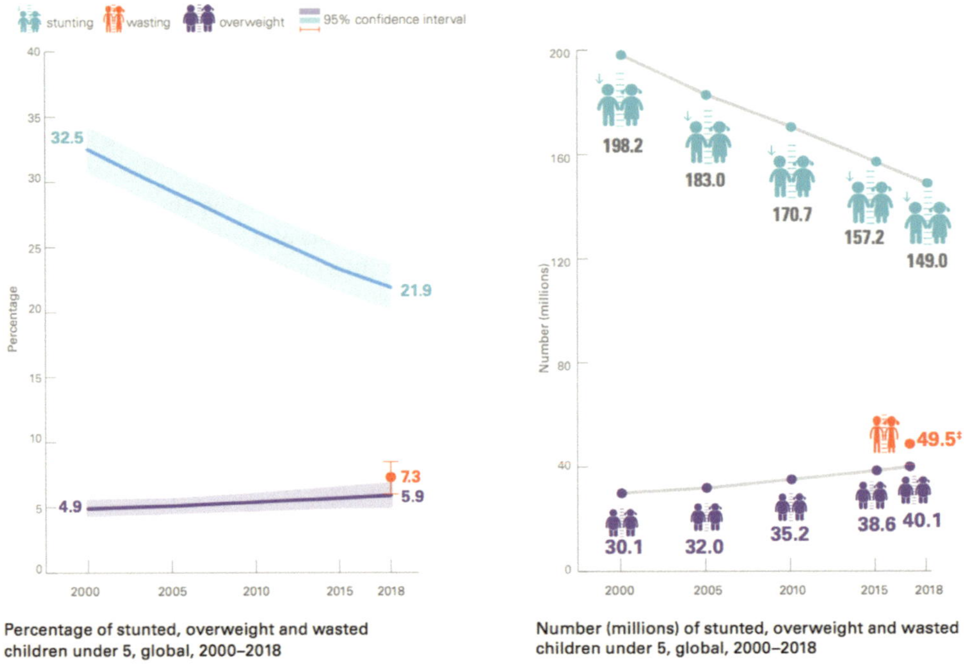

Figure 2.
Trends in global burden of malnourished under-5 children [8].

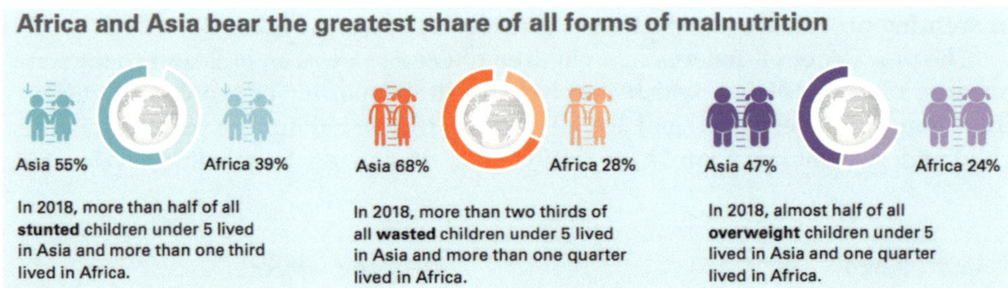

Figure 3.
Comparison of burden of malnourished under-5 Asian and African children [8].

Goals (SDG) 2 focuses on end hunger, achieves food security and improves nutrition and promotes sustainable agriculture. By 2030, end all forms of malnutrition, including achieving, by 2025, the internationally agreed targets on stunting and wasting in children under 5 years of age, and address the nutritional needs of adolescent girls, pregnant and lactating women and older persons and indicators are primarily prevalence of stunting, wasting and overweight among children under 5 years of age. In a recently released Global Nutrition Report 2018, revealed the prevalence of stunting, wasting and overweight at national level as 37.9, 20.8 and 2.4% respectively [10].

In India as per National Family Health Survey IV (2014–2015, recent in the series) 38.4, 21 and 35.7% of children below 5 years suffer from stunting, wasting and underweight respectively (corresponding figure for NFHS III, 2005–2006 were 47.9, 19.8 and 42.5% respectively). Prevalence of severe acute malnutrition (SAM) in India is 7.5% [11]. Trends in various nutritional indicator values and U5 mortality rate from 2000 to 2018 (India) are shown in **Figure 5**.

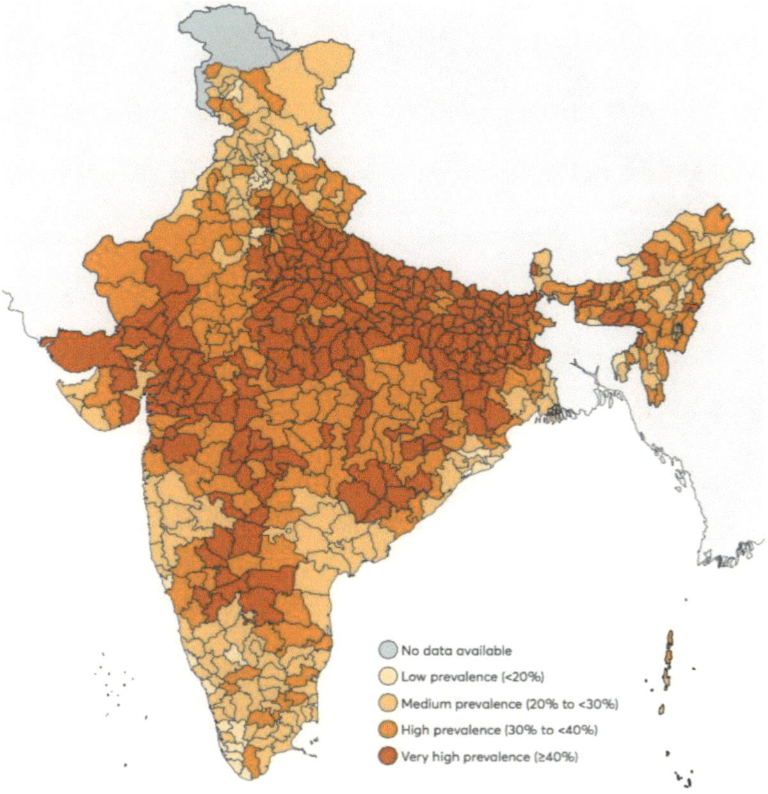

Figure 4.
Pattern of stunting prevalence among Indian districts (source: Menon et al. 2018).

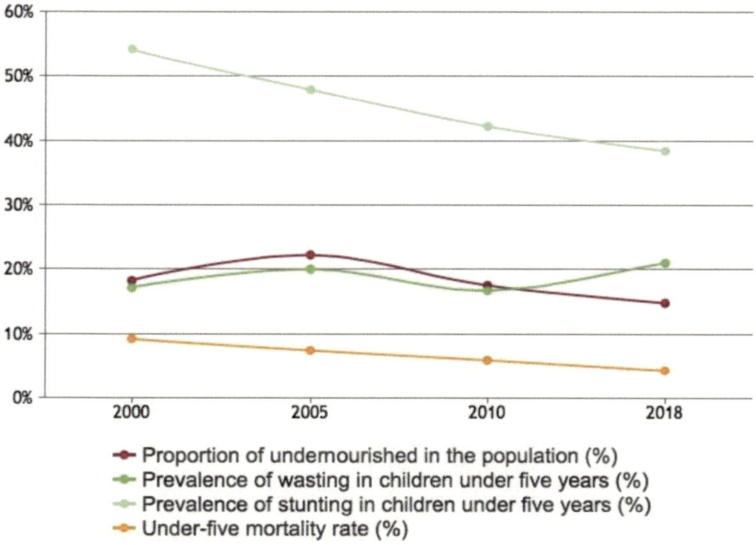

Figure 5.
Trends in various nutritional indicator values and U5 mortality rate from 2000 to 2018 (India).

In the 2018 Global Hunger Index, India ranks 103rd out of 119 qualifying countries [12]. With a score of 31.1, India suffers from a level of hunger that is serious. **Figure 6** depicts dimensions and indicators of Hunger index and its relationship with child malnutrition.

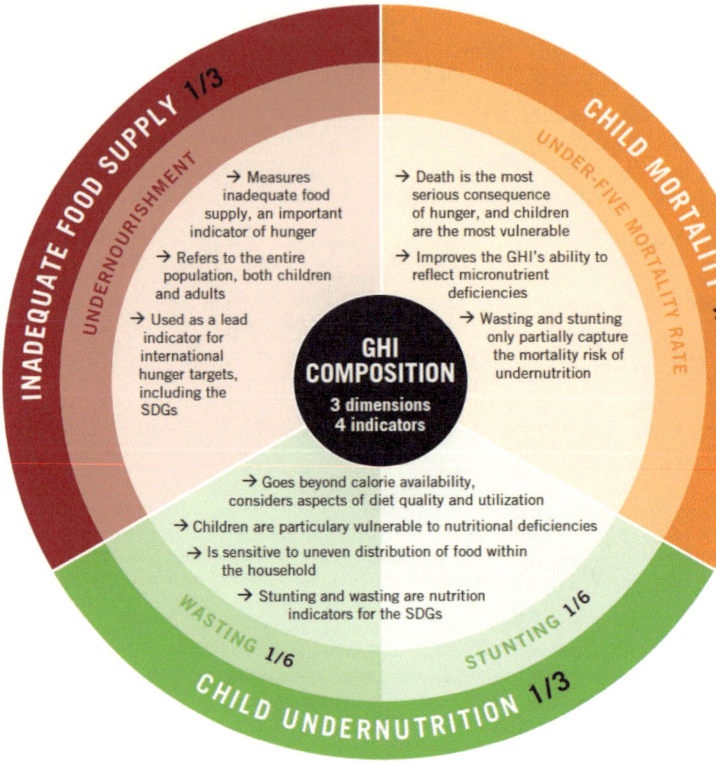

Figure 6.
Diagrammatic representation of child undernutrition with Hunger Index.

8. Web of factors maintaining malnutrition in Indian communities

'Asian enigma' is a phenomenon of persistent and unusually high prevalence of child undernutrition in South Asia as compared to countries at similar levels of income or economic growth. In-depth analysis into why malnutrition is so resistant to improvement shows its complex aetiology. The immediate causes of undernutrition reflect a negative synergy between inadequate food intake and repeated infectious diseases. Underlying these causes is a constellation of factors particularly salient to India [13]. These include especially poor sanitation and high rates of open defecation that leads to various kinds of infestations, infections and environmental enteropathy; poor coverage of health services and half-hearted implementation of nutritional programs and policies; no political commitment and will, and economic, social determinants including economic growth and income distribution, deficiencies in governance and strategic leadership and the status of women [14, 15].

A new study from Harvard Chan School of Public Health has now pinpointed the five top risk factors responsible for more than two-thirds of the problem. Short maternal stature, extreme poverty, poor dietary diversity and mother's lack of education are among the top five risk factors for malnutrition in children in India. Examining an array of 15 well-known risk factors for chronic undernutrition among children in India, the study found that the five top risk factors were essentially markers of poor socioeconomic conditions as well as poor and insecure nutritional environments in children's households [16].

Economic conditions definitely play a crucial role. On the one hand, money is required to look after food, water and sanitary living conditions, whereas on the other hand, approximately 22% of the Indian population live below the poverty line. Rural population, a major chunk (especially agriculturists) is mostly dependent on rains for their income. They always live in a state of uncertainty of income. Apart of income, illiteracy plays a crucial role. Most of the people are not aware about their health, nutrition, balanced diet and breastfeeding practices. Without these, effective nutrition communication campaign cannot succeed in their purpose.

India ranked 97 among a list of 118 countries on hunger as per Global Hunger Index (GHI). It concludes that Indian population does not have access to sufficient and nutritious food. National Food Security Act is a great step in the direction of ensuring greater access to adequate quantity of quality food at affordable cost via Targeted Public Distribution System (PDS). Desired outcomes were not achieved due to corruption in PDS [17]. Wastage of food grains (theft, rotting) in Food Corporation of India (FCI) warehouses has also dented the access of food to common man. Greater efforts are needed to strengthen the existing initiatives to make them as corruption free and efficient institutions to get better results.

State of maternal health illiteracy is an important determinant of child nutritional status. The type of care a mother provides to her child depends to a large extent on her knowledge and understanding of some aspects of basic nutrition and health care [18].

Millions of beneficiaries have benefitted by ICDS Scheme however, problems are being observed in ensuring supply of quality food, and its uniform distribution. Anganwadi Workers (AWWs) and Anganwadi Helpers (AWHS) at Anganwadi centres are often dissatisfied by low wages. Thus they fail to play an effective role in tackling the problem of malnutrition.

8.1 Scam in ICDS project unearthed

Dibrugarh, Assam: two organizations have brought charges of rampant corruption in the Integrated Child Development Scheme (ICDS) amounting to more than Rs. 37 lakh in Panitola ICDS project of the district. While the officer-in-charge of the ICDS project in Panitola development block has drawn the money for 2007–2008 through two cheques (Nos. 107,895 and 017896) from UCO Bank, Dibrugarh after collecting the cheque from the district social welfare department, All India Youth Federation and All Assam Mottock Yuba Chatra Sanmilan unearthed through Right to Information (RTI) Act that the money has not been utilized till date. Suspecting misuse of the allotted money, the two organizations have demanded that the district administration institute an enquiry into the anomaly immediately. They have also demanded exemplary punishment on the erring officials (source: The Assam Tribune, 12 May 2008).

Village Health, Sanitation and Nutrition committee (VHSNC), one of the key elements of the National Rural Health Mission are non-functional in many of the states due to lack of funds. Similarly, Village Child Development Centres (VCDCs) were set up by state government of Maharashtra to provide malnourished children with medical care and nutritious meals. These centres are mostly non-functional due to lack of funds [19].

8.2 Toffees in the name of nutritious food

In Nigoha, the hot food scheme has stopped functioning due to lack of funds. The condition of Rampura AWC is also the same. The centre does not open on regular basis. The AWH, Sarvesh Kumari, distributes toffees instead of proper nutritional food to the limited number of children who come to the centre. Villagers are not even aware of the facilities provided to them by the AWC. Community participation is also lacking as parents do not sent their children to the centres (source: Dainik Jagran, Lucknow, 1 November 2009).

Social and cultural factors may also affect malnutrition. State government of Uttar Pradesh launched Hausla Poshan Yojana in 2016 to combat malnutrition among mothers and children by providing food cooked by Anganwadi Workers. Surprisingly beneficiaries refused to consume food because lower caste people prepared it [20]. Upper caste community considers lower caste as untouchables. Another cultural practice still prevalent in Indian communities is child marriage that is acting as limiting factor in improving health of children. 27% of girls in India are married before their 18th birthday and 7% are married before the age of 15. According to UNCIEF, India has the highest absolute number of child brides in the world [21]. A weak mother is likely to give birth to a weak child. This maintains the cycle of undernourishment.

As discussed earlier that poor sanitation is directly linked to malnourished children. The Census 2011 told us only 32% of India's rural households had toilets. 59% of the 1.1 billion people in the world who practice open defecation live in India. On 2 October 2014, Swachh Bharat Mission was launched throughout country with an aim to achieve the vision of a 'Clean and Open Defecation-Free India' by 2 October 2019 [22]. These targets are difficult to achieve, as implementation is poor, as observed from the slow progress in meeting the targets, and the existence of several newly constructed but non-functional toilets [21, 23].

Diarrheal disease kills an estimated 300,000 children less than 5 years of age (13% deaths in this age-group) in India each year. Most mortality related to diarrhoea occurs in less developed countries, and the highest rates of diarrhoea occur among malnourished children under-1. The case fatality rate is highest among children aged 6–12 months because at this age the immune system is not yet fully mature, maternal antibodies are waning, and the foods introduced to complement breastfeeding may be contaminated. Among children who survive severe diarrhoea, chronic infections can contribute to malnutrition. In turn, malnutrition makes children vulnerable to diarrhoea infections. Better access to clean water and sanitation is the key, with fewer weak and malnourished children becoming infected [24, 25].

9. Commitments and targets to track progress to end malnutrition

Recognizing the seriousness of malnutrition for global health, in 2012 and 2013, the member states of the World Health Organization (WHO) adopted a series of targets to significantly reduce the burden of many of these forms of malnutrition by 2025 (**Table 1**).

Progress to tackle all forms of malnutrition remains unacceptably slow. The 2018 Global Nutrition Report [10] tracks country progress against the following global

Child health goals under NHP-2017 and SDG-2030

Child health indicator	Current status	NHP 2017	SDG 2030
Neonatal mortality rate (NMR)	24	16 by 2025	<12
Infant mortality rate (IMR)	34	28 by 2019	—
Under-5 mortality rate (U5MR)	39	23 by 2025	≤25

Source: Ref. [33]

Table 1.
Global nutrition targets 2025 [12].

targets: child overweight, child wasting, child stunting, exclusive breastfeeding, diabetes among women, diabetes among men, anaemia in women of reproductive age, obesity among women and obesity among men. Data for 194 countries was analysed. As per this report, India is listed among those countries, which are on track for none (zero) of the nine targets. The key driver behind the goal to reach Zero Hunger and malnutrition is to ensure that no one is left behind in the pursuit of food and nutrition security. In the Indian context, this will also mean greatly improving the health of women and children.

10. Determinants of child malnutrition

The causes of malnutrition in India are several and multifaceted, from direct factors to underlying contributors. Malnutrition in children occurs as a complex interplay among various factors like socio-demographic, maternal, gender, home environment, dietary practices, hand washing and other hygiene practices, etc. **Figure** 7 depicts factors significantly associated with malnutrition among under-5 children in India.

Socio-economic and demographic factors: literacy status of parents especially mother's education, caste, birth order of child, gender of household head, residence,

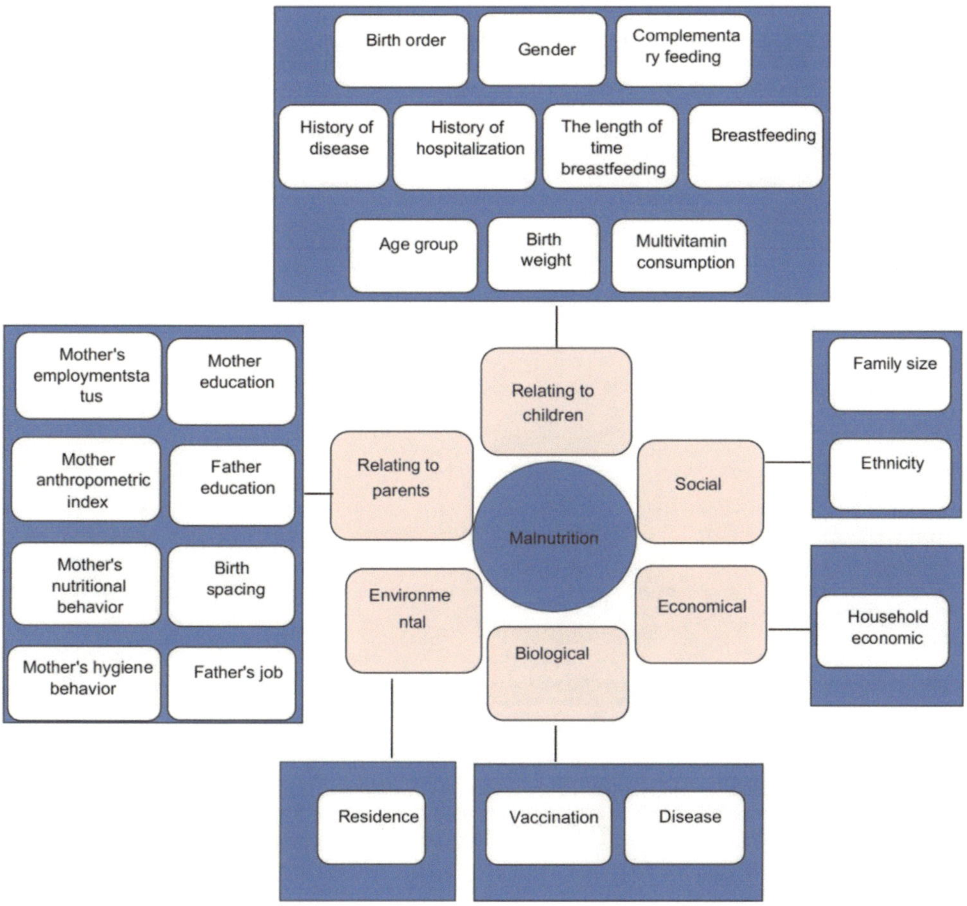

Figure 7.
Factors significantly associated with malnutrition among under-5 children [36].

type of house, type of family (single/joint) lower socio-economic status, poverty, food insecurity, etc. are such important factors.

Gender: female gender is vulnerable to severe forms of malnutrition across all ages due to socio-cultural factors (responsible for child bearing and rearing, last one to consume food in the family). Undernourished girls grow up to become undernourished women who give birth to a new generation of undernourished children [26].

Maternal factors: short stature, mother's nutrition, mother's age, antenatal and natal care, infections, smoking and exposure to second hand smoke are important maternal factors.

Breastfeeding practices: inadequate, insufficient, inappropriate breastfeeding practices lay down foundation of malnutrition. Breastfed children are protected from infections in better way than who are not breastfed. Early initiation of breastfeeding and right timing of initiation of complementary feeding are also quite important [27].

Home environment: large family size, food insecurity, toilet facility, sanitation and hygiene practices, water storage and handling practices are extremely important factors.

Open air defecation: open defecation, the practice of people defecating out in the open wherever it is convenient, is one of the main factors leading to malnutrition. Approximately in the urban setting, 12% of the population open defecate and rural areas that number is 72%. Open defecation leads to polluted water; up to 75% of India's surface water is polluted.

Poor hand hygiene: role of hand hygiene is quite important in prevention of infections and thereby malnutrition. Availability of soap and water is an important

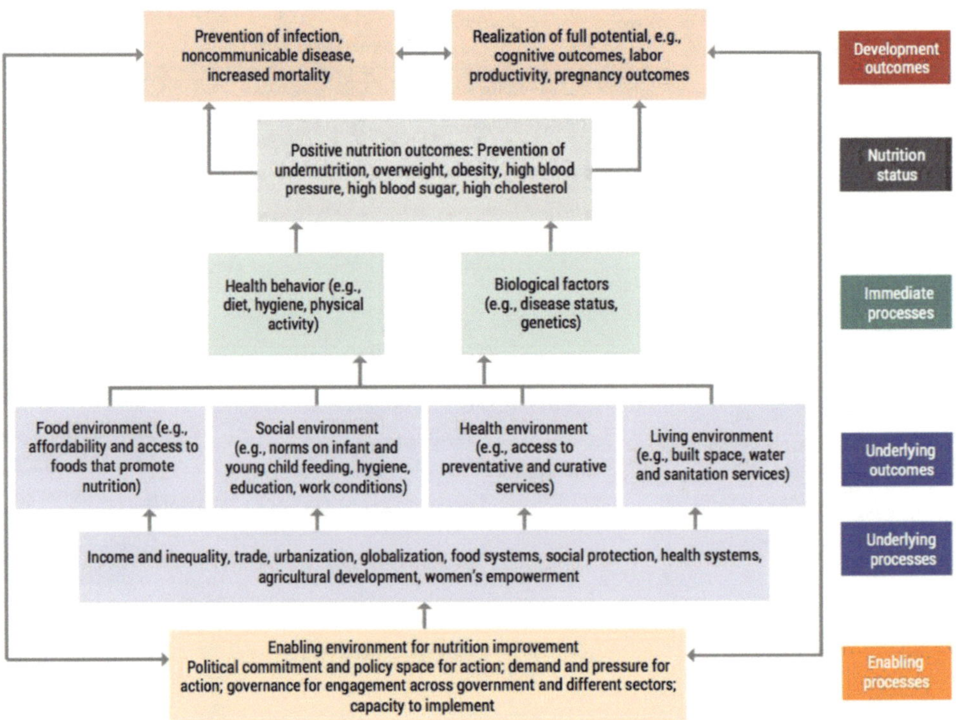

Figure 8.
Underlying drivers of malnutrition (source: Reproduced from the Global Nutrition Report 2016. International Food Policy Research Institute. 2016. Global Nutrition Report 2016: From promise to impact: Ending malnutrition by 2030. Washington, DC).

determinant. Hand washing before preparation, serving and eating meals and after going to toilets can prevent malnutrition to a great extent.

Diarrhoeal disease: diarrhoea is a leading cause of malnutrition in children under 5 years old. Poor sanitation, lack of access to clean water and inadequate personal hygiene are responsible for an estimated 88% of childhood diarrhoea in India. Based on current evidence, washing hands with soap can reduce the risk of diarrheal diseases by 42–47%. A survey conducted by UNICEF in 2005 on well-being of children and women had shown that only 47% of rural children in the age-group 5–14 wash hands after defecation [28].

Figure 8 depicts the underlying drivers of malnutrition. They are complex and multidimensional which include inter alia poverty, inequality and discrimination. Control of malnutrition will require a comprehensive approach targeting all these causes and contributors across sectors and stakeholders.

11. The life-course approach on malnutrition

The challenge of malnutrition calls for a multidisciplinary approach that targets multiple underlying factors. Crucial stages in people's lives have particular relevance for their health, and the life-course approach recognizes the same. Taking a life-course perspective to tackle malnutrition emphasizes its intergenerational effects.

Intervening in the preconception period is fundamental to improve nutritional status and health behaviours in young people and adolescents and to prevent the transmission of risk to the next generation. Adopting a combination of top-down approaches through policy initiatives and bottom-up engagement of key stakeholders such as young people is recommended to prevent malnutrition over the first 1000 days of life. Targeting pregnancy and preconception periods increases nutrition awareness and influences dietary habits.

It is an established fact that preventing undernutrition during the first 1000 days of a child's life, i.e. from conception to the second birthday is quite important. This time period is very precious because child may not be able to grow to her or his full potential in the future and even irreversible damage may occur, if foundation for good nutrition is not properly established during this time period. However it does not mean that there are no other entry points to improve nutrition. Moreover, even with coverage of 90% of direct nutrition interventions, only 20% of stunting deficits would be addressed [29]. It is essential that preconception services are incorporated into a continuum from childhood to antenatal care, involving both partners and linked to interventions to promote school attendance in young girls, and the planning of first and subsequent pregnancies [30].

The life course approach underlines the dynamic nutritional needs at different stages of life, this holds true especially with women. It also explains that at each stage of life, nutrition can and should be addressed in order to break the cross-generational cycle of malnutrition [31].

Figure 9 depicts the life course approach which explains how the first 1000 days are critically important. Investments in nutrition must extend as per the changing needs and risks at later stages in life, such as adolescent girls and women of reproductive age. It also points towards underlying causes of malnutrition and the need to address them. Underlying causes can only be satisfactorily addressed with intersectoral co-ordination and involvement like health, agriculture, water and sanitation, social protection and education. These sectors should be involved taking into account the specific needs and roles of women in order to work towards sustainable and inclusive solutions.

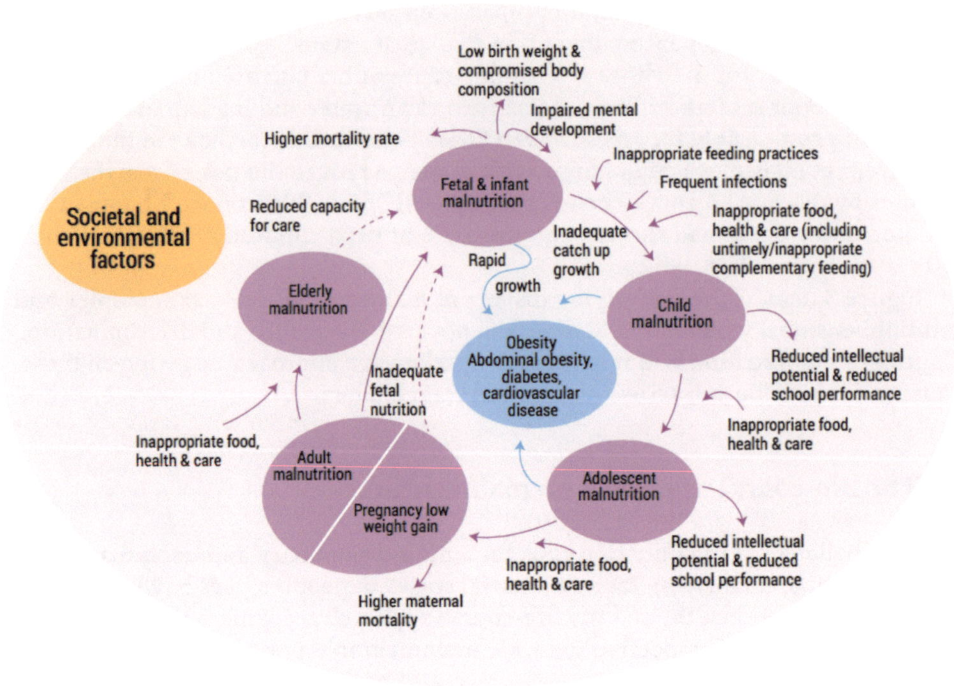

Figure 9.
The life-course approach on malnutrition.

12. The fight against malnutrition

Massive and strategic investments have been made to combat malnutrition by governments of various countries, India being one of them. Recently (in April 2016), the United Nations General Assembly adopted a resolution proclaiming the UN Decade of Action on Nutrition from 2016 to 2025. The Decade aims to catalyse policy commitments that result in measurable action to address all forms of malnutrition. The aim is to ensure all people have access to healthier and more sustainable diets to eradicate all forms of malnutrition worldwide. Sustained and concrete results can only be achieved only if determinants of malnutrition are addressed with holistic approach [32].

Outcomes of these nutritional interventions are evident in the declining patterns in some of the India's key health variables as reported by National Family Health Surveys NFHS-3 (2005–2006) and NFHS-4 (2015–2016) data.

12.1 Data on nutrition indicators as per the last available national survey (NFHS 4)

- 38% of children below 5 years (urban: 31%, rural: 41%) are stunted (low height for age).
- 21% (urban: 20%, rural: 22%) are wasted (low weight for height).
- 36% (urban: 29%, rural: 38%) are underweight (low weight for age).
- More importantly, 7.5% of children are suffering from severe acute malnutrition, as per the last available national survey.

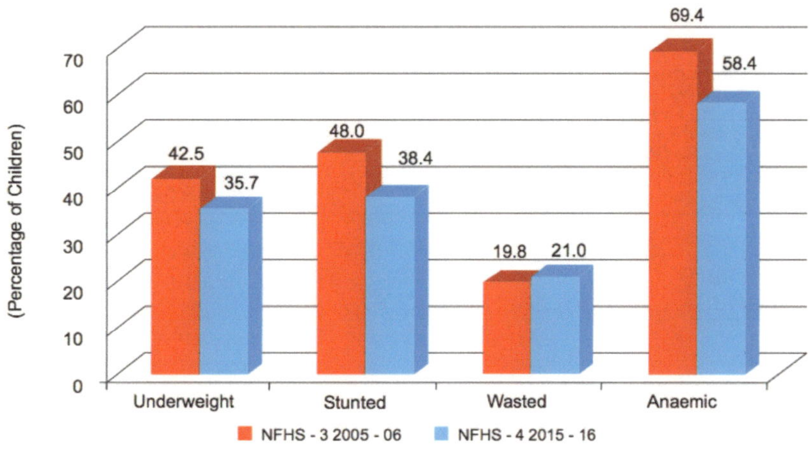

Figure 10.
Comparison of nutrition indicators as per NFHS-3 and NFHS-4 (source: NFHS-4, 2015–2016. Note: data on anaemia pertain to children aged 6–59 months).

12.2 Related indicators

- Only 41.6% newborns initiated on breastfeeding within 1 hour of birth while 54.9% children breastfed exclusively till 6 months of age.
- Complementary feeding started for only 42.7% children on time (more than 6 months of age).
- 58.4% of children in age group 6–59 months are anaemic.

Figure 10 shows the comparison of nutrition indicators as per NFHS-3 and NFHS-4.

12.3 Status of child mortality in India

- The U5MR has declined at a faster pace in the period 2008–2016, registering a compound annual decline of 6.7% per year, compared to 3.3% compound annual decline observed over 1990–2007 [33].
- As per latest Sample Registration System, 2016 Report; The U5MR in India is 39/1000 live births, IMR is 34/1000 live births and NMR is 24/1000 live births. This translates into an estimated 9.6 lakh under-5 child deaths annually.
- Four States together contribute to 56% of all child deaths in the country, namely-Uttar Pradesh (2.45 lakhs), Bihar (1.2 lakhs), Madhya Pradesh (1.0 lakh) and Rajasthan (0.75 lakh).
- About 46% of under-five deaths take place within the first 7 days of birth, 62% within first 1 month of birth.

The state of malnutrition in India is alarming and disturbing. A lot of work has been done, progress has been made but definitely pace of improvement is too slow. Following table shows the current status of important child health indicators and time bound targets to be achieved under National Health policy and Sustainable Development Goals (SDGs).

Child health goals under NHP-2017 and SDG-2030			
Child health indicator	**Current status**	**NHP 2017**	**SDG 2030**
Neonatal mortality rate (NMR)	24	16 by 2025	<12
Infant mortality rate (IMR)	34	28 by 2019	—
Under-5 mortality rate (U5MR)	39	23 by 2025	≤25

Source: Ref. [33]

Table 2.
Targets for child mortality in India.

Sustainable Development Goals (SDGs) were released by the UN in 2016 (till 2030) showing unfinished agenda of Millennium Development Goals (MDGs) ended in 2015. SDG 2 calls to end hunger, achieve food security and improved nutrition and promote sustainable agriculture whereas SDG 3 calls to ensure healthy lives and promote well-being for all at all ages (**Table 2**).

13. Policy level nutritional interventions to fight against malnutrition

Based on understanding towards a wide range of factors responsible for malnutrition among children, the policy called for the adoption of a multi-sectoral approach along with multiple measures to achieve the goal of optimum nutrition for all. Important government led policy level interventions and programmes to combat malnutrition are as follows:

13.1 Direct policy measures

a. Inclusion of all vulnerable groups (children, adolescent girls, mothers, expectant women) under the safety cover of ICDS.

b. Fortification of essential food items with legal provisions (e.g. twin fortification of salt with both iodine and iron).

c. Popularize low cost nutritious food.

d. Control of micro-nutrient deficiencies with special focus on vulnerable groups.

13.2 Indirect policy measures

a. Guarantee of food security to citizens by increasing production of food grains.

b. Improve dietary pattern by promoting production and increasing per capita availability of nutritionally rich food.

c. Prevention of food adulteration by law.

d. Strengthening nutrition surveillance.

e. Improving purchasing power of landless, rural and urban poor.

f. Improving public distribution system (PDS).

The Government of India enacted the National Food Security Act (NFSA) in 2013 to enable food and nutritional security by ensuring access to adequate quantity of quality food at affordable prices to people to live a life with dignity. This legal provision has put the onus on the state to guarantee basic entitlements.

13.3 Plans, programmes and missions

a. Mid-day Meal Programme, 1962–1963

b. Goiter Control Programme, 1962 (now known as National Iodine Deficiency Disorders Control Programme)

c. Special Nutrition Programme, 1970–1971

d. Balwadi Nutrition Programme, 1970–1971

e. Nutritional Anaemia Prophylaxis Programme, 1970

f. Prophylaxis Programme against Blindness due to Vitamin A Deficiency, 1970

g. Integrated Child Development Services (ICDS), 1975

h. National Diarrhoeal Diseases Control Programme, 1981

i. Wheat-based Supplementary Nutrition Programme, 1986

j. National Plan of Action on Nutrition, 1995

k. Public Distribution System, 1997

l. The National Population Policy (NPP) 2000

m. The National Health Policy 2002

n. National Nutrition Mission, 2003

o. National Health Mission (NRHM—2005–2017)

p. National Health Mission, 2013 (subsumes former Rural and Urban Health Missions) National Iron+ Initiative, 2013

q. Promotion of Infant and Young Child Feeding Practices Guidelines, 2013

r. Weekly Iron and Folic Acid Supplementation, 2015

s. National Deworming Day, 2015

t. Sustainable Development Goals (2016–2030)

u. New National Health Policy, 2017

v. Establishment of: Nutritional Rehabilitation Centres; Village Health Sanitation & Nutrition Committee

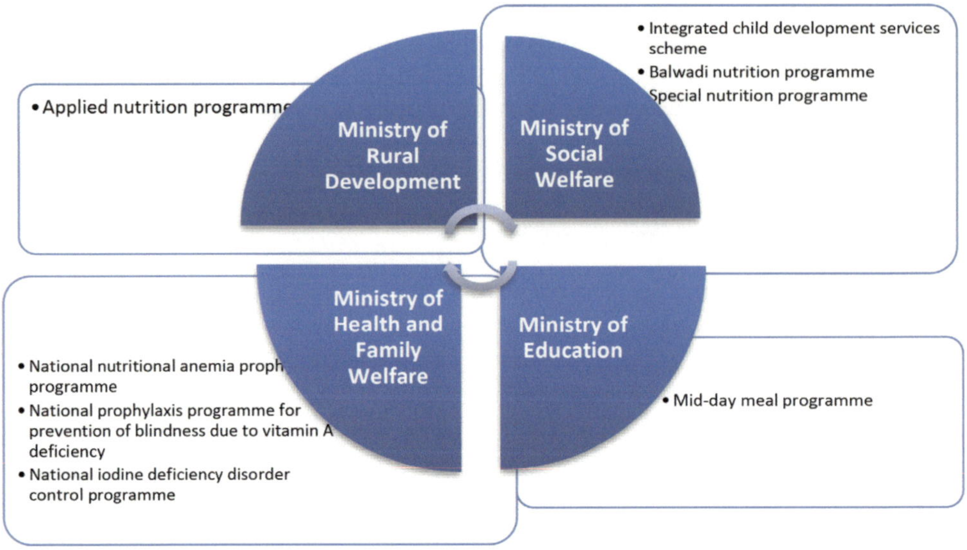

Figure 11.
Multi ministerial involvement showing political commitment and intersectoral approach to end malnutrition.

w. Bi-annual Vitamin-A Supplementation

x. Village Health & Nutrition Days (at Anganwadi centres)

y. Reproductive, Maternal, Newborn, Child and Adolescent (RMNCH+A) Strategy

Figure 11 depicts multi ministerial involvement showing political commitment and intersectoral approach to end malnutrition.

14. Strategic nutrition related interventions rolled out by government of India

Various community nutritional programmes are running in India to combat child malnutrition and to get nutrition on track. These are based on strategic nutrition related interventions. A few of them are discussed below.

Promotion of Infant and Young Child feeding practices (IYCF): exclusive breastfeeding for first 6 months, complementary feeding beginning at 6 months and appropriate infant and young child feeding practices (IYCF) are being promoted. Mother's Absolute Affection (MAA) programme was launched in 2016 to promote breastfeeding and infant feeding practices by building the capacity of frontline health workers and comprehensive IEC campaign.

Establishment of Nutritional Rehabilitation Centres (NRCs): NRCs have been set up at facility level to provide medical and nutritional care to Severe Acute Malnourished (SAM) children under 5 years of age who have medical complications. In addition, the mothers are also imparted skills on child care and feeding practices so that the child continues to receive adequate care at home.

Anaemia Mukt Bharat (AMB): to address anaemia, NIPI has been launched which includes provision of supervised bi-weekly Iron Folic Acid (IFA) supplementation by ASHA for all under-5 children, weekly IFA supplementation for 5–10 years old children and annual/biannual De-worming. The AMB strategy—Intensified Iron Plus Initiative—aims to strengthen the existing mechanisms and foster newer strategies of tackle anaemia, focused on six target beneficiary groups, through six interventions and six institutional mechanisms; to achieve the envisaged target under the POSHAN Abhiyaan. The strategy focuses on testing & treatment of anaemia in school going adolescents and pregnant women using newer technologies, establishing institutional mechanisms for advanced research in anaemia, and a comprehensive communication strategy including mass/mid media communication material.

National De-worming Day (NDD): recognising worm infestation as an important cause of anaemia, National Deworming Day (NDD) is being observed annually on 10th February targeting all children in the age group of 1–19 years (both school enrolled and non-enrolled).

Biannual Vitamin A Supplementation is being done for all children below 5 years of age.

Village Health and Nutrition Days (VHNDs) are also being organized for imparting nutritional counselling to mothers and to improve child care practices.

A few schemes and services rendered by them are tabulated (**Table 3**) below as per target group.

14.1 NGO's working to combat malnutrition

- Akshaya Patra—the world's largest NGO-run mid-day meal programme serving wholesome school lunch to over 1.76 million children in 15,668 schools across 12 states in India.
- Avantha Foundation Fighting malnutrition in Bihar
- Nutrition CINI India
- Salaam Baalak Trust Health and Nutrition
- The Hunger Project India—The Hunger Project
- Cry NGO in India to Support Child Rights
- CARE India
- Save the Children India
- Feeding India works to eradicate hunger, malnutrition and food wastage in India
- Yashoda Foundation
- SNEHA—Society for nutrition
- Freedom From hunger India trust
- FMCH India—Foundation for Mother and Child Health
- Real Medicine Foundation
- *Indian Impact*—It offers individuals and corporations an easy way to help improve their nearest Anganwadi centre, and supports NGOs that are working to reduce malnutrition.

Target group	Schemes	Major services from schemes
Children (0–3 years)	ICDS	ICDS: supplementary nutrition, growth monitoring, counselling health education of mothers on child care, promotion of infant and young child feeding, home based counselling for early childhood stimulation, referral and follow up of undernourished and sick children.
	RCH-II, NRHM	NRHM: home-based new born care, immunization, micronutrient supplementation, deworming, health check-up, management of childhood illness and severe under-nutrition, referral and cashless treatment for first month of life. Care of sick newborns, facility-based management of severe acute malnutrition and follow up.
	Rajiv Gandhi National Creche Scheme	Rajiv Gandhi National Creche Scheme: support for the care of children of working mothers.
Children (3–6 years)	ICDS	ICDS: non-formal preschool education, growth monitoring, supplementary nutrition, referral, health education and counselling for care givers.
	RCH-II, NRHM	NRHM: immunization micronutrient supplementation, deworming, health check-up, management of illnesses and severe undernutrition
	Rajiv Gandhi National Creche Scheme	Rajiv Gandhi Creche Scheme: support for care of children of working mothers
	Total Sanitation Campaign (TSC)/Nirmal Bharat Abhiyan (NBA)	TSC/NBA: household-level sanitation facilities
	National Rural Drinking Water Programme (NRDWP)	NRDWP: availability of safe drinking water
School going children (6–14 years)	Mid-Day Meals (MDM),	Mid-day meal: hot cooked meal to children attending school.
	Sarva Shiksha Abhiyan (SSA)	SSA: support knowledge dissemination on nutrition by inclusion of Nutrition related topics in syllabus and curriculums for formal education, school health check-up, mid-day meal.

Table 3.
Selected nutritional schemes and services rendered as per target group.

15. Case study

The following case study from Tamil Nadu, a southern state of India focuses on the complex challenges faced and the progress made so far as part of efforts towards combating malnutrition. It also demonstrates how lessons are being learned along the way.

15.1 The Tamil Nadu integrated nutrition project (TINP)

The Tamil Nadu Integrated Nutrition Project (TINP), a World Bank assisted intervention program in rural south India, offered nutrition and health services to children under-5 and pregnant and lactating women. TINP-I (1980–1989) eventually covered 174 blocks. It was a forerunner of the Bangladesh Integrated Nutrition

Project (BINP). TINP-II (1991–1997) covered all non-ICDS blocks in the Tamil Nadu state. TINP-II was replaced by World Bank assisted ICDS III (WB-ICDS III) from 1998.

Since 1975, Indian government is providing a package of services to combat child hunger and malnutrition under Integrated Child Development Services (ICDS) program through Anganwadi centres (AWCs). Anganwadi means 'courtyard shelter' in local language.

15.2 TINP I (1980–1989)

Approximately 1.25–2.40% points per year (ppt/year) drop in underweight prevalence was noted among beneficiaries. On comparing drop in underweight prevalence between TINP areas and non-TINP areas, it was noticed that drop was approximately 0.83–1.12 ppt/year in TINP areas whereas reduction in underweight prevalence was approximately 0.26–1.12 ppt/year in non-TINP areas.

At the same duration, reduction in the underweight prevalence was estimated as 0.7 ppt/year for the whole of India. Therefore it can be stated that quarter to half of the reduction in underweight prevalence was attributable to the TINP project.

Having achieved a significant reduction in severe early childhood malnutrition, TINP-1 became inspiration for others as a 'success story' during the 1980s. Evaluations indicated a decrease in underweight prevalence of about 1.5% points per year in participating districts, twice the rate in non-participating districts. Several factors contributed in the success story of TINP I viz. selective feeding (the careful focus on supplementing the dietary intake of young children when their growth faltered and until their growth resumed), clarity in job responsibilities and description, positive worker-supervisor ratio and robust monitoring system.

15.3 TINP II (1990–1997)

TINP II was rolled out to move beyond reducing severe malnutrition and with a more ambitious objective to significantly reduce the burden of moderate malnutrition. In other words, it shifted towards a more preventive focus. Core strategies adopted in TINP II were regular growth monitoring, nutrition education, health check-ups, supplementary feeding of malnourished children and growth-faltering children, high-risk pregnant and lactating women.

Approximately 6.0 ppt/year drop in underweight prevalence was noted among TINP II beneficiaries. It was also noticed that drop was approximately 1.1 ppt/year in TINP areas. As per estimates of World Bank, the current underlying trend in the state was to be 5.0–7.0 ppt/year, which is most certainly an overestimate.

In the nutshell, TINP II achieved its objective to decrease severe malnutrition but failed to achieve its objective for moderate malnutrition.

A few lessons were learned from TINP II before planning a next phase nutritional intervention. For example, need to work on localized capacity building, improved home-based care by intensifying community mobilization and targeted interpersonal communications, and feeding of 6–24 months old children. Next phase of nutritional programme must incorporate improved service delivery, supportive counselling of caregivers, social mobilization and participatory learning.

Take home massage from TINP I was, interventions that are targeted using nutritional criteria, integrated within a broader health system and effectively supervised and managed can significantly reduce severe malnutrition. TINP II taught us that going further and preventing children from becoming moderately malnourished is in many ways a tougher task, and demands a significant shift in strategy [34, 35].

16. Conclusion

The facts and discussion presented above, highlights the worrying unacceptably high prevalence and universality of malnutrition in all its forms in Indian communities, but it is both preventable and treatable. Beyond health, malnutrition is also impacting the social and economic development. In Indian context, poverty, maternal health illiteracy, LBW, diseases like diarrhoea, home environment, dietary practices, hand washing and poor hygiene practices are few important factors responsible for very high prevalence of malnutrition. Government of India has rolled out various community nutritional programmes to combat malnutrition and to get nutrition on track. Despite enormous challenges, India has made considerable progress in tackling hunger and undernutrition in the past two decades, yet this pace of change has been unacceptably slow, uneven and many have been left behind. But with sustained prioritization, increased resource allocation, adopting comprehensive, coordinated and holistic approach with good governance and help of civil society, India has the potential to end malnutrition in all its forms and turn the ambition of the Sustainable Development Goals into a reality for everyone.

Author details

Abhishek Singh
Department of Community Medicine, SHKM Government Medical College, Haryana, India

*Address all correspondence to: abhishekparleg@gmail.com

References

[1] Blössner M, de Onis M. Malnutrition: Quantifying the Health Impact at National and Local Levels. WHO Environmental Burden of Disease Series, No. 12. Geneva: World Health Organization; 2005

[2] Thang NM, Popkin BM. In an era of economic growth, is inequity holding back reductions in child malnutrition in Vietnam? Asia Pacific Journal of Clinical Nutrition. 2003;**12**:405-410

[3] HUNGaMA: Fighting hunger and malnutrition: The HUNGaMA Survey Report. 2011. Available from: https://www.eldis.org/document/A72128

[4] World Bank. India's Undernourished Children: A Call for Reform and Action. 2019. Available from: http://web.worldbank.org/WBSITE/EXTERNAL/COUNTRIES/SOUTHASIAEXT/0,contentMDK:20916955~pagePK:146736~piPK:146830~theSitePK:223547,00.html [Accessed: 05 March 2019]

[5] Global Panel. The Cost of Malnutrition: Why Policy Action is Urgent. 2016. Available from: https://glopan.org/sites/default/files/pictures/CostOfMalnutrition.pdf

[6] Rice AL, Sacco L, Hyder A, Black RE. Malnutrition as an underlying cause of childhood deaths associated with infectious diseases in developing countries. Bulletin of the World Health Organization. 2000;**78**:1207-1221

[7] Sengupta P, Philip N, Benjamin AI. Epidemiological correlates of under-nutrition in under-5 years children in an urban slum of Ludhiana. Health and Population; Perspectives and Issues. 2010;**33**(1):1-9

[8] UNICEF-WHO-World Bank: Joint Child Malnutrition Estimates – 2019 edition. Available from: https://data.unicef.org/topic/nutrition/malnutrition/

[9] Nelson GC, Rosegrant MW, Koo J, Robertson R, Sulser T, Zhu T, et al. Impact on Agriculture and Costs of Adaptation. Washington DC: International Food Policy Research Institute (IFPRI); 2009

[10] Global Nutrition Report. 2018. Available from: https://globalnutritionreport.org/reports/global-nutrition-report-2018/

[11] National Family Health Survey IV. 2015-2016. Available from: http://rchiips.org/NFHS/NFHS-4Reports/India.pdf

[12] The Global Hunger Index. 2018. Available from: https://www.globalhungerindex.org/about/

[13] Gragnolati M, Shekar M, Gupta MD, Bredenkamp C, Lee YK. India's Undernourished Children: A Call for Reform and Action. Washington DC: The International Bank for Reconstruction and Development/The World Bank; 2005

[14] Black RE, Allen LH, Bhutta ZA, Caulfield LE, De Onis M, Ezzati M, et al. Maternal and child Undernutrition study group. Maternal and child undernutrition: Global and regional exposures and health consequences. The Lancet. 2008;**371**(9608):243-260

[15] Victora CG, Adair L, Fall C, Hallal PC, Martorell R, Richter L, et al. Maternal and child undernutrition study group. maternal and child undernutrition: Consequences for adult health and human capital. The Lancet. 2008;**371**(9609):340-357

[16] Harvard TH. Chan School of Public Health. Top Risk Factors for Child Undernutrition in India identified. 2017. Available from: https://www.hsph.harvard.edu/news/press-releases/top-risk-factors-for-child-undernutrition-in-india-identified/

[17] Leakage and Corruption in India's Public Distribution System. 2016. Available from: https://www.isid.ac.in/~epu/acegd2016/papers/Daniel Overbeck.pdf

[18] Mishra VK, Retherford RD. Women's education can improve child nutrition in India. National Family Health Survey Bulletin. 2000;**15**:1-4

[19] Rapid Assessment of RKS and VHSNC in Sikkim. Available from: http://www.rrcnes.gov.in/study_report/Final%20RKS%20-%20VHSNC%20Assessment%20Report%20130217.pdf

[20] Preventing Hunger and Malnutrition in India. 2017. Available from: https://www.orfonline.org/research/preventing-hunger-and-malnutrition-in-india/

[21] UNICEF. Child-Marriage. 2019. Available from: https://unicef.in/Whatwedo/30/Child-Marriage

[22] Swachh Bharat Survey. Swachhta Status in India, July–December 2017. Available from: http://www.mospi.gov.in/sites/default/files/publication_reports/Final_Report_Swachha_Status_India_16oct18.pdf

[23] Swachhta Status Report. Most of Rural India Still Opts for Open Defecation: National Sample Survey (NSS) Report. 2016. Available from: http://upsccivilservices.com/news_update/662/Most_of_rural_India_still_opts_for_open_defecation_NSS_report

[24] Caulfield LE, de Onis M, Blossner M, Black RE. Under nutrition as an underlying cause of child deaths associated with diarrhea, pneumonia, malaria and measles. The American Journal of Clinical Nutrition. 2004;**80**:193-198

[25] Bhutta ZA, Ahmed T, Black RE, Cousens S, Dewey K, Giugliani E, et al. What works? Interventions for maternal and child undernutrition and survival. The Lancet. 2008;**371**(9610):417-440

[26] Griffiths P, Matthews Z, Hinde A. Gender, family, and the nutritional status of children in three culturally contrasting states of India. Social Science and Medicine. 2002;**55**:775-790

[27] Victora CG, Bahl R, Barros AJ, França GV, Horton S, Krasevec J, et al. Breastfeeding in the 21st century: Epidemiology, mechanisms, and lifelong effect. The Lancet. 2016; **387**(10017):475-490

[28] Lakshminarayanan S, Jayalakshmy R. Diarrheal diseases among children in India: Current scenario and future perspectives. Journal of Natural Science, Biology, and Medicine. 2015;**6**(1):24

[29] Bhutta ZA, Das JK, Rizvi A, Gaffey MF, Walker N, Horton S, et al. Maternal and child nutrition study group. Evidence-based interventions for improvement of maternal and child nutrition: What can be done and at what cost? The Lancet. 2013;**382**(9890): 452-477

[30] Kuruvilla S, Sadana R, Montesinos EV, et al. A life-course approach to health: Synergy with sustainable development goals. Bulletin of the World Health Organization. 2018; **96**(1):42-50

[31] Jacob CM, Hanson M. A life-course approach for influencing policies to prevent childhood malnutrition. Crisis and Opportunity of the Double Burden. 2018;**2016**(2025):18

[32] de Onis M, Blössner M. The World Health Organization global database on child growth and malnutrition: Methodology and applications. International Journal of Epidemiology. 2003;**32**:518-526

[33] SRS Statistical Report 2016. Office of the Registrar General and Census Commissioner, India. Ministry of Home Affairs, Government of India. 2016.

Available from: http://www.censusindia.gov.in/vital_statistics/SRS_Reports__2016.html

[34] Gillespie S, Haddad L. The Double Burden of Malnutrition in Asia: Causes, Consequences, and Solutions. New Delhi: Sage Publications India; 2003

[35] Essential Nutrition Actions: Improving Maternal, Newborn, Infant and Young Child Health and Nutrition. Geneva: World Health Organization; 2013. Annex 3, Nutrition Programme Case Studies. Available from: https://www.ncbi.nlm.nih.gov/books/NBK258728/

[36] Mohseni M, Aryankhesal A, Kalantari N. Factors associated with malnutrition among under five-year-old children in Iran: A systematic review. Annals of Tropical Medicine and Public Health. 2017;**10**:1147-1158

Section 3

Dehydration

Chapter 3

Dehydration

Fatihi Hassan Soliman Toaimah and Fysel Manthattil

Abstract

Dehydration is one of the common presentations to the general practice or emergency departments (EDs) in children having acute gastroenteritis (AGE). Assessing the severity of dehydration remains a challenge among physicians, and the dehydration scales currently available are inaccurate. The correct assessment of dehydration is the basis for proper management of acute diarrhea in children. Rapid oral rehydration therapy (ORT) over 3–4 hours remains the cornerstone treatment of AGE with dehydration. It is advisable to reserve intravenous (IV) rehydration therapy for patients with severe dehydration and for those who fail ORT. Rapid standard-volume (20 ml/kg/hour) IV bolus of isotonic solution for 1–4 hours followed by oral fluid intake or maintenance IV fluids seems to be adequate for most cases requiring IV rehydration. A minority of patients may be presented with complications due to diarrheal dehydration, such as dyselectrolytemia, which requires careful calculation of fluids and electrolytes with slow correction approach.

Keywords: gastroenteritis, dehydration, children, rehydration, pediatric, diarrhea

1. Introduction

Dehydration is the main clinical manifestation and the most frequent complication in pediatric patients with AGE. It remains to be a common reason for ED visits, and it can lead to significant morbidity and mortality rates [1]. Management of gastroenteritis is based mainly on the proper assessment of dehydration severity and correction of dehydration.

2. Body water distribution

In newborn babies, 75–80% of the total body weight constitutes the total body water (TBW) (varies with the gestational age), which decreases to 67% of body weight (2/3) after the neonatal period. There is a further decrease that reaches 60% by the end of the first year, and this percentage remains the same during the rest of life. After puberty and in adulthood, TBW is 60% in males and 55% in females. The TBW is divided into two components throughout the body: intracellular fluid compartment (ICF), which constitutes 40% of TBW, and extracellular fluid (ECF), which forms the remaining 20%. The ECF comprises interstitial fluid (IF) (15% of the TBW), and the remaining 5% of the TBW comprises intravascular plasma (**Figures 1** and **2**) [2–4]. This distribution of body fluids can have an impact on the management of pediatric gastroenteritis, as most of the fluid loss in AGE comes from the ECF. This matters because ECF contains a lot of sodium (135–145 mEq), and ICF contains a lot of potassium (150 mEq). In a brief duration of illness

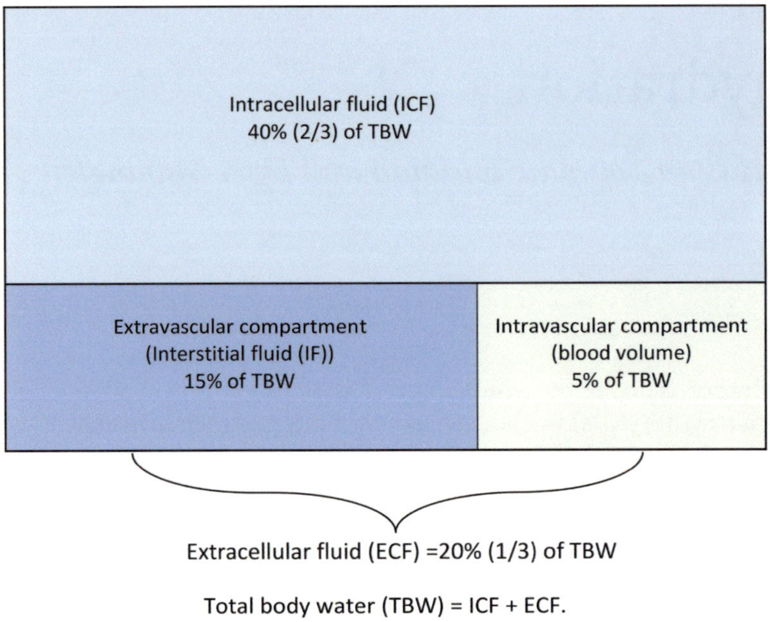

Figure 1.
The percentage distribution of body fluids in the various compartments in a 1-year-old infant [2].

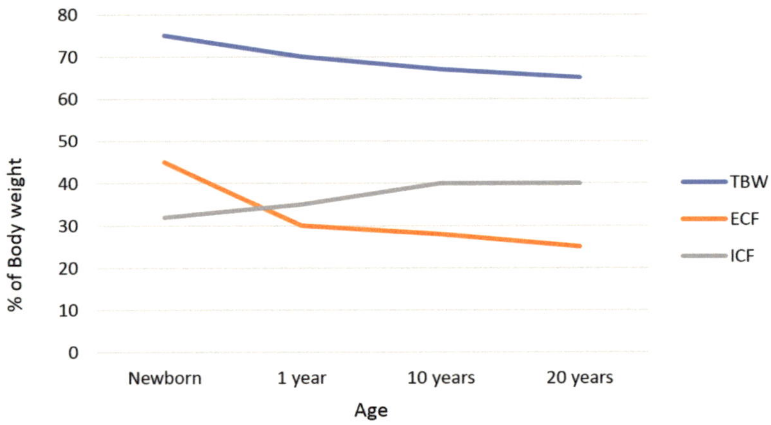

Figure 2.
Body water compartments in relation to age [2–4].

(<3 days), 80% of the deficit is typically from the ECF. After more than 3 days of illness, the deficit from the ECF decreases to 60%. Fluid losses for longer than 7 days are equally lost from ECF (50%) and ICF (50%) [5].

3. Assessment of dehydration

Accurate and quick assessment of the degree of dehydration is important for proper treatment and disposition of infants and children with AGE [6]. The percentage of weight loss is the best measure to assess the degree of dehydration, as shown in Eq. (1). However, this method is impractical because in most patients the pre-illness weight is not known [7].

$$\% \ of \ dehydration = \frac{[(pre - illness \ weight \ in \ kg) - (illness \ weight \ in \ kg)] \times 100}{pre - illness \ weight \ in \ kg} \quad (1)$$

3.1 Clinical assessment of dehydration

Current validated dehydration scales may help in assessing the versatile presentations of dehydration more objectively. Most of them illustrate clinical signs that can be assessed easily and rapidly, which can facilitate stratification of patients into dehydration categories. There are three clinical scales designed to estimate dehydration severity in children below 5 years of age: the World Health Organization (WHO) scale (**Table 1**), the Gorelick scale (**Table 2**), and the Clinical Dehydration Scale (CDS) (**Table 3**) [8–10].

Using common tools to evaluate and assess dehydration would be more helpful in day-to-day practice. Consistent evidence supports the CDS which is more useful and easy to use in assessing dehydration. This scale in combination with other criteria should be used to guide the proper medical interventions in individual

Characteristics	No dehydration	Some dehydration (>1 sign)	Severe dehydration (>1 sign)
Alertness	Well, alert	Irritable or drowsy	Lethargic or poorly responsive
Eyes	Normal	Sunken	Sunken
Thirst	Drinks normally	Drinks eagerly	Poor or weak drinking
Skin turgor	Goes back quickly	Goes back slowly (<2 s)	Return very slowly (>2 s)

Table 1.
WHO scale for dehydration in children aged 1 month–5 years old.

Characteristics	No or minimal dehydration	Moderate-to-severe dehydration
General appearance	Alert	Restless, lethargic, unconscious
Capillary refill	Normal	Prolonged or minimal
Tears	Present	Absent
Mucous membranes	Moist	Dry, very dry

Table 2.
Gorelick (4-item) scale for dehydration in children aged 1 month–5 years. Scoring: ≥2 clinical signs indicates ≥ 5% loss of body weight from baseline (moderate dehydration), and ≥3 clinical signs indicates ≥ 10% loss of body weight from baseline (severe dehydration). The presence of two or more of these signs had a sensitivity of 79% and a specificity of 87% in predicting 5% dehydration.

Characteristics	Score of 0	Score of 1	Score of 2
General appearance	Normal	Thirsty, restless, or lethargic but irritable when touched	Drowsy, limp, cold, sweaty ± comatose
Eyes	Normal	Slightly sunken	Very sunken
Mouth and tongue	Moist	Sticky	Dry
Tears	Present	Decreased	Absent

Table 3.
Clinical dehydration scale (CDS) for children aged 1 month–3 years. Scoring: ≥2 clinical signs indicates ≥ 5% loss of body weight from baseline (moderate dehydration), and ≥3 clinical signs indicates ≥ 10% loss of body weight from baseline (severe dehydration). The presence of two or more of these signs had a sensitivity of 79% and a specificity of 87% in predicting 5% dehydration.

cases [11]. Clinical dehydration scales are imprecise and of limited diagnostic value in children with gastroenteritis [12]. As a screening test of dehydration, historical points are moderately sensitive. Classification of dehydration into NO, SOME, and SEVERE are recommended by WHO and other groups [1, 8].

Prolonged capillary refill time, abnormal skin turgor, and abnormal respiratory pattern still remain the best three individual examination signs for assessment of dehydration. Increased capillary refill time was the strongest individual sign as an isolated finding to predict dehydration, and the poor predictor of dehydration was reduced urine output. Combinations of signs perform much better than individual signs. History taking and laboratory tests show limited utility [13].

3.2 Laboratory assessment of dehydration

Blood biochemistry is generally not accurate and not routinely required for assessment of dehydration. Commonly done laboratory tests such as blood urea nitrogen (BUN) and bicarbonate concentrations are generally helpful only when the results are markedly abnormal. A normal serum bicarbonate concentration of more than 15 or 17 mEq/L appears to be valuable in reducing the likelihood of dehydration. These laboratory tests done for assessing dehydration should not be considered definitive, which could be reserved for children requiring IV fluids and suffering from severe dehydration, altered conscious state or convulsions, suspected hypernatremia, suspicion of hemolytic uremic syndrome and children with pre-existing medical conditions that predispose to electrolyte abnormalities [14, 15]. Historical points and laboratory tests only have limited utility for assessing dehydration [10]. Laboratory investigations should be performed if the results will influence the management and outcome of a specific patient.

4. Management of dehydration

Oral rehydration should be the first line of treatment for pediatric gastroenteritis with intravenous (IV) fluid therapy being used if the oral route fails [16, 17].

4.1 Oral rehydration therapy (ORT)

Oral rehydration is the preferred method for replacing fluid and electrolyte deficits resulting from dehydration secondary to acute gastroenteritis. ORT is a safe, easy-to-use, efficacious, and cost-effective alternative to intravenous rehydration for uncomplicated gastroenteritis in children [18].

The use of ORT is based on the principle of glucose-facilitated sodium transport across the intestinal mucosa. The ORT facilitates the absorption of water and sodium for the compensation of fluid losses. Additionally, the absorption can be adequate for the replacement of significant fluid loss, such as in cholera. The absorption of potassium and bicarbonate is maintained by the osmotic gradient in the intercellular space. Metabolic acidosis, usually associated with dehydration, can be safely corrected by this mechanism. The currently available ORT contains an appropriate amount of sodium, glucose, and other electrolytes and is of appropriate osmolality to maximize clinical efficacy [19].

The WHO, Centers for Disease Control (CDC), and the American Academy of Pediatrics (AAP) all support the use of ORT for some (mild–moderate) dehydration [8, 20, 21]. Rapid ORT in mild dehydration is done by giving 50 ml/kg over 4 hours. For moderate dehydration, 100 ml/kg can be given over the same duration. Generally, children being enterally rehydrated do not require blood tests.

4.2 Ondansetron to facilitate ORT

Children who received oral ondansetron initially were less likely to be administered IV rehydration compared with those given placebo. In addition, both oral and IV ondansetron administration are associated with reduced rate of hospitalization [17]. Ondansetron is contraindicated in children with long QT syndrome, concomitant drugs that prolong QT, and to be used cautiously in children with heart disease.

4.3 Discharge criteria

Children can be discharged home when the following levels of recovery are achieved: satisfactory rehydration status as shown by clinical improvement, IV or NG fluids not required, and no significant losses. Adequate family education, proper instructions, and medical follow-up should be provided.

4.4 Patient/parent education

Inform about the expected natural course of the illness, prevention of transmission and looking at signs of dehydration. Encourage breastfeeding continuation in small babies, early refeeding, and the correct method of preparing ORS. Educate about the importance of giving anti-rotavirus vaccination and of course not to use unnecessary medication in simple AGE.

4.5 Other rehydration methods

Nasogastric route is a safe rehydration technique with minimal adverse effects which has been adequately studied. Many clinical trials showed this method to have similar efficacy compared to IV therapy. Rapid NG rehydration using gastrolyte, 50 ml/kg for fluid deficit replacement over 4 hours, appears to be appropriate for children with mild-to-moderate dehydration [22]. If nasogastric rehydration is required beyond 4 hours, check urea and electrolyte concentration (UEC) and blood glucose level (BGL), and reassess the patient for hydration status.

4.6 Intravenous (IV) rehydration

Intravenous rehydration should be reserved for patients with severe dehydration or shock and for those with some (mild-to-moderate) dehydration who fail ORT. Fluid containing not less than 0.9% sodium chloride is preferred for rehydration [23, 24]. Using hypotonic fluids predisposes for dilutional hyponatremia due to excess antidiuretic hormone (ADH) secretion in children with AGE. Serum electrolytes and BGL are required in children with severe dehydration and/or requiring IV fluid therapy for correction of dehydration.

The WHO recommends IV rehydration to be rapidly completed over 3–4 hours [8]. Rapid replacement of ECF improves gastrointestinal and renal perfusion, allowing earlier oral intake and a faster correction of electrolyte and acid-base abnormalities, which results in excellent recovery rate and decreased length of stay in ED [25].

4.6.1 Resuscitation

Resuscitate shock/near shock with a prompt intravenous infusion of 20 ml/kg of 0.9% sodium chloride solution or Ringer's lactate solution as fast as possible. Reassessing and repeating boluses given, as necessary, are required until the patient is recovered from shock and then followed by maintenance IV fluids [26].

4.6.2 Rapid standard-volume IV rehydration

The clinical standard is to administer 20 mL/kg/h of isotonic crystalloid fluid, such as 0.9% normal saline or lactated Ringer's solution. Reassess the patient after each bolus, and if the patient is still dehydrated, a total of 2–4 fluid boluses may allow rapid restoration of intravascular volume which can bring rapid recovery. Rapid IV rehydration followed by oral fluids is adequate for initial rehydration for most patients requiring IV fluid therapy. For those refusing oral intake, continuous infusion of maintenance IV fluids are to be given until oral fluids are tolerated [27]. Glucose solution should be added once ECF volume has been restored and addition of potassium considered once the child passes urine and serum electrolytes are known [28].

4.6.3 Rapid large-volume IV rehydration

Refer to the correction of dehydration using a large volume of fluids over a relatively shorter time (50–60 ml/kg/hour). Ultra-rapid IV rehydration may be associated with electrolyte abnormalities and longer hospital stay or delayed discharge and therefore is not recommended [29, 30].

Children with acute watery diarrhea and severe dehydration, such as cholera, who fail ORT, can benefit from large-volume IV rehydration (100 ml/kg) of Ringer's lactate solution or normal saline over 3–6 hours. Frequent reassessment is required, and if hydration status is not improving, IV fluids should be given more rapidly [31]. Further research investigations are needed to justify the use of rapid large-volume IV rehydration in pediatric gastroenteritis.

5. Electrolyte disturbances

Dyselectrolytemia is a serious complication of AGE with dehydration. The majority of electrolyte disorders associated with AGE in children can be adequately treated using ORT.

5.1 Hypernatremia (serum sodium > 145 mmol/L)

Hypernatremia leads to hypertonicity that can be potentially dangerous as there is a greater likelihood of neurological manifestations. Most frequently, it is due to water deficit from increased water losses in diarrhea and due to reduced water intake during the illness.

As in any type of dehydration, the primary aim should be restoration of hemodynamic stability by administration of isotonic fluids. The gradual replacement of water deficit remains the gold standard treatment for hypernatremic dehydration [32]. The recent advance in management of hypernatremia is to give isotonic (0.9% sodium chloride + 5% glucose) than hypotonic solution to correct the calculated fluid deficit slowly. The more the solution contains free water, the higher the risk of developing hyponatremia during rehydration [23, 33].

5.2 Hyponatremia (serum sodium < 135 mmol/L)

It represents an excess of water in relation to sodium in ECF [34]. Hyponatremia is seldom symptomatic unless the serum Na is <120 or if the hyponatremia occurs quickly [35]. Hyponatremia may be presented with nausea, vomiting, headache, irritability, lethargy, confusion, muscle cramps, convulsions, disorientation, and reduced consciousness and places the patient at risk of neurologic impairment [36].

The initial goal in treating hyponatremia is the restoration of intravascular volume with isotonic saline and to be followed by a slower correction using 0.9% sodium chloride + 5% glucose. In severe hyponatremia or symptomatic children, the goal is to raise the serum sodium to 120–125 mmol/L or until the seizure stops [35]. As a rule of thumb, IV infusion of 3% NaCl, 3–5 ml/kg over 15–30 min, will raise serum Na by 5 mEq/L.

6. Systematic approach to a child with AGE and dehydration: summary of the assessment and management of AGE with dehydration in children

See **Figure 3**.

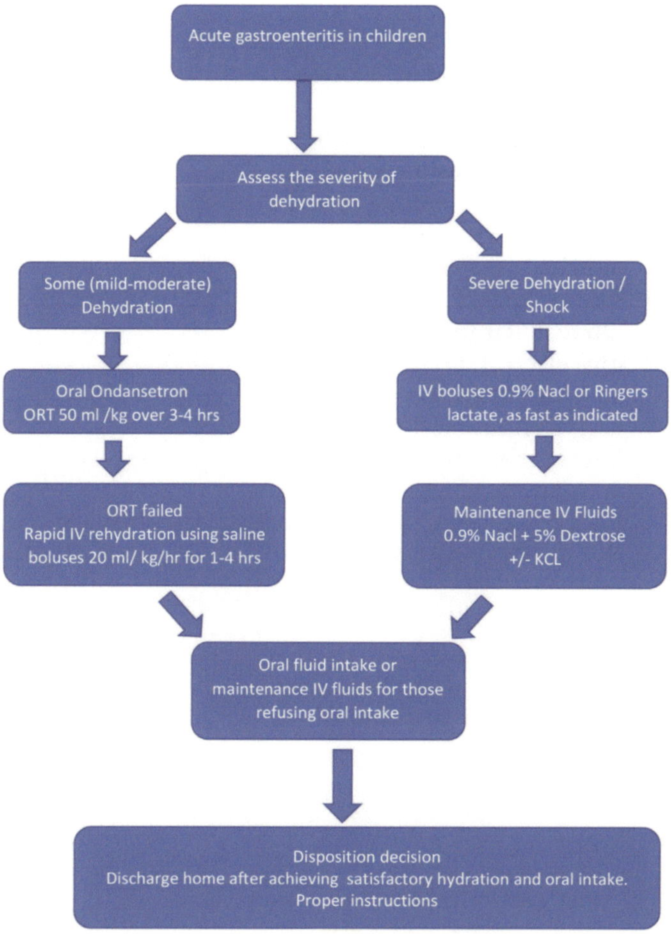

Figure 3.
Flow chart for the management of pediatric gastroenteritis with dehydration.

7. Conclusions

The management of a child with a dehydrating gastroenteritis requires careful initial assessment and reassessment of hydration status. The majority of gastroenteritis in infants and children are simple and can be treated by ORT. In children who presented with severe dehydration or those with some dehydration and fail ORT, IV rehydration is required. Rapid IV rehydration using standard boluses of isotonic fluids followed by oral fluid intake or maintenance IV fluids for those refusing oral intake appears sufficient for most patients requiring IV fluids. Patients achieving satisfactory hydration status and tolerating oral intake can be discharge home with proper instructions.

Acknowledgements

The authors thank physicians and nurses staff who are working at the Pediatric Emergency center (PEC) Alsadd, Hamad Medical Corporation (HMC), Qatar, for their help and support.

Conflict of interest

The authors declare no conflict of interest.

Acronyms and abbreviations

AGE	acute gastroenteritis
TBW	total body water
ECF	extracellular fluid
ICF	intracellular fluid
UEC	urea electrolyte concentration
BGL	blood glucose level
ORT	oral rehydration therapy
IV	intravenous
ADH	antidiuretic hormone
NICE	National Institute for Health and Care Excellence
ED	emergency department

Author details

Fatihi Hassan Soliman Toaimah[1,2]* and Fysel Manthattil[1]

1 Department of Pediatrics, Pediatric Emergency Medicine, Hamad Medical Corporation, Doha, Qatar

2 Department of Clinical Pediatrics, Weill Cornell Medical College, Doha, Qatar

*Address all correspondence to: fsoliman2@yahoo.com

References

[1] King CK, Glass R, Bresee JS, Duggan C, Centers for Disease Control and Prevention. Managing acute gastroenteritis among children: Oral rehydration, maintenance, and nutritional therapy. MMWR—Recommendations and Reports. 2003;**52**(RR-16):1-16

[2] Jain A. Body fluid composition. Pediatrics in Review. 2015;**36**:141-152. DOI: 10.1542/pir.36-4-141

[3] O'Brien F, Walker IA. Fluid homeostasis in the neonate. Pediatric Anesthesia. 2014;**24**:49-59

[4] Schmidt GL. Fluids and electrolytes. In: Corkins M, editor. The ASPEN Pediatric Nutrition Support Core Curriculum. Silver Spring, MD: American Society for Parenteral and Enteral Nutrition; 2010. pp. 87-102

[5] Gamble JL. Chemical Anatomy, Physiology and Pathology of Extracellular Fluid. Cambridge, MA: Harvard University Press; 1951, Fig 36–A

[6] Colletti JE, Brown KM, Sharieff GQ, Barata IA, Ishimine P. The management of children with gastroenteritis and dehydration in the emergency department. The Journal of Emergency Medicine. 2010;**38**:686-698

[7] Roberts KB. Fluid and electrolytes: Parenteral fluid therapy. Pediatrics in Review. 2001;**22**:380-387. DOI: 10.1542/pir.22-11-380

[8] World Health Organization. The Treatment of Diarrhoea. A Manual for Physicians and Other Senior Health Care Workers. 4th rev ed. Geneva, Switzerland: World Health Organization; 2005. Available from: http://whqlibdoc.who.int/publications/2005/9241593180.pdf

[9] Gorelick M, Shaw K, Murphy K. Validity and reliability of clinical signs in the diagnosis of dehydration in children. Pediatrics. 1997;(5):e1-e6

[10] Parkin PC, Macarthur C, Khambalia A, Goldman RD, Friedman JN. Clinical and laboratory assessment of dehydration severity in children with acute gastroenteritis. Clinical Pediatrics. 2010;**49**:235-239

[11] Pringle K, Shah SP, Umulisa I, et al. Comparing the accuracy of the three popular clinical dehydration scales in children with diarrhea. International Journal of Emergency Medicine. 2011;**4**:58. DOI: 10.1186/1865-1380-4-58

[12] Falszewska A, Dziechciarz P, Szajewska H. Diagnostic accuracy of clinical dehydration scales in children. European Journal of Pediatrics. 2017;**176**:1021-1026. DOI: 10.1007/s00431-017-2942-8

[13] Steiner MJ, DeWalt DA, Byerley JS. Is this child dehydrated? Journal of the American Medical Association. 2004;**291**(22):2746-2754

[14] Vega RM, Avner JR. A prospective study of the usefulness of clinical and laboratory parameters for predicting percentage of dehydration in children. Pediatric Emergency Care. 1997;**13**:179-182

[15] Yilmaz K, Karabocuoglu M, Citak A, Uzel N. Evaluation of laboratory tests in dehydrated children with acute gastroenteritis. Journal of Paediatrics and Child Health. 2002;**38**:226-228

[16] Hartling L, Bellemare S, Wiebe N, Russell K, Klassen TP, Craig W. Oral versus intravenous rehydration for treating dehydration due to gastroenteritis in children (review). Evidence-Based Child Health. 2007;**2**:163-218. DOI: 10.1002/ebch.121

[17] Freedman SB, Adler M, Seshadri R, Powell EC. Oral ondansetron for gastroenteritis in a pediatric emergency department. The New England Journal of Medicine. 2006;**354**(16):1698-1705

[18] Canavan A, Arant BS. Diagnosis and management of dehydration in children. American Family Physician. 2009;**80**(7):692-696

[19] Fontaine O. Multicentre evaluation of reduced-osmolarity oral rehydration salts solution. International study group on reduced-osmolarity ORS solutions. Lancet. 1995;**345**:282-285

[20] Centers for Disease Control and Prevention. Guidelines for the Management of Acute Diarrhea after a Disaster. 2014. Available from: https://www.cdc.gov/disasters/disease/diarrheaguidelines.html

[21] American Academy of Pediatrics. Statement of endorsement: Managing acute gastroenteritis among children; oral rehydration, maintenance, and nutritional therapy. Pediatrics. 2004;**114**:507. DOI: 10.1542/peds.114.2.507

[22] National Institute for Health and Care Excellence (NICE). Diarrhoea and vomiting caused by gastroenteritis: Diagnosis, assessment and management in children younger than 5 years. In: Clinicalguideline. Vol. 84. 2009. Available from: www.nice.org.uk/guidance/cg84

[23] Friedman JN, Beck CE, DeGroot J, Geary DF, Sklansky DJ, Freedman SB. Comparison of isotonic and hypotonic intravenous maintenance fluids: A randomized clinical trial. JAMA Pediatrics. 2015;**169**(5):445-451. DOI: 10.1001/jamapediatrics.2014.3809

[24] Neville KA, Verge CF, Rosenberg AR, O'Meara MW, Walker JL. Isotonic is better than hypotonic saline for intravenous rehydration of children with gastroenteritis: A prospective randomised study. Archives of Disease in Childhood. 2006;**91**(3):226-232

[25] Levy JA, Bachur RG. Intravenous dextrose during outpatient rehydration in pediatric gastroenteritis. Academic Emergency Medicine. 2007;**14**:324-331

[26] Fleisher GR, Ludwig S, Henretig FM. Textbook of Pediatric Emergency Medicine: Shock. 5th ed. Philadelphia: Lippincott Williams and Wilkins; 2006

[27] Guarino A, Ashkenazi S, Gendrel D, Lo Vecchio A, Shamir R, Szajewska H. European society for pediatric gastroenterology, hepatology, and nutrition/european society for pediatric infectious diseases evidence-based guidelines for the management of acute gastroenteritis in children in Europe: Update 2014. Journal of Pediatric Gastroenterology and Nutrition. 2014;**59**(1):132-152. DOI: 10.1097/MPG.0000000000000375

[28] Reid SR, Losek JD. Rehydration: Role for early use of intravenous dextrose. Pediatric Emergency Care. 2009;**25**:49-52

[29] Iro MA, Sell T, Brown N, Maitland K. Rapid intravenous rehydration of children with acute gastroenteritis and dehydration: A systematic review and meta-analysis. BMC Pediatrics. 2018;**18**(1):44. DOI: 10.1186/s12887-018-1006-1

[30] Toaimah FH, Mohammad HM. Rapid intravenous rehydration therapy in children with acute gastroenteritis: A systematic review. Pediatric Emergency Care. 2016;**32**(2):131-135. DOI: 10.1097/PEC.0000000000000708

[31] World Health Organization. 3 Diarrhoea and dehydration. In: Manual for the Health Care of Children in Humanitarian Emergencies. Geneva: World Health Organization; 2008.

Available from: https://www.ncbi.nlm.nih.gov/books/NBK143745/

[32] Finberg L. Hypernatremic (hypertonic) dehydration in infants. The New England Journal of Medicine. 1973;**289**:196-198. DOI: 10.1056/NEJM197307262890407

[33] Powers KS. Dehydration: Isonatremic, hyponatremic, and hypernatremic recognition and management. Pediatrics in Review. 2015;**36**(7):274-285. DOI: 10.1542/pir.36-7-286

[34] Sawaya RD, Ravandi B. Fluids and Electrolyte Management. AHC; 2016. Available from: https://www.ahcmedia.com/articles/137306-fluids-and-electrolyte-management-part-fluids-dehydration-and-sodium-homeostasis

[35] Madden MA. Paediatric Fundamental Critical Care Support. 2nd ed. Illinois, USA: Society of Critical Care Medicine; 2013. pp. 8-9

[36] Meyers RS. Pediatric fluid and electrolyte therapy. Journal of Pediatric Pharmacology and Therapeutics. 2009;**14**:204-211

Section 4

Treatment

Chapter 4

Current Knowledge and Therapeutic Strategies of Herbal Medicine for Acute Diarrhea

Muhammad Akram, Muhammad Daniyal, Aatiqa Ali, Iftikhar Ahmed Khan, Rida Zainab, Khan Usmanghani and Wei Wang

Abstract

Diarrhea is a common gastrointestinal problem characterized by loose watery stool and mild to severe dehydration. Annually, about 1.7–5 billion new cases of diarrhea were reported. In developing countries, it is more common, where young kids have diarrhea approximately three times/year. In 2013, 1.26 million deaths occurred due to diarrhea, whereas in 1990, the figure was slightly higher (2.58 million). In 2012, diarrhea was the second most common reason of death (11%, n = 0.76 million) in children less than 5 years. Although various synthetic drugs are being prescribed as standard therapy for diarrhea, they have side effects. It is possible to prescribe the herbal medicine for diarrhea, which is safe and effective. In this study, medicinal plants discussed are proven to be scientifically active in diarrheal diseases. This study reviews about current medicinal plants used in the treatment of diarrhea. The use of medicinal plants for diarrhea results in improvement of the symptom. Moreover, studies on large scale are needed to characterize the beneficial role of medicinal plants in the treatment of diarrhea.

Keywords: diarrhea, infectious disease, medicinal plants, efficacy, literature review

1. Introduction

Diarrhea increased the frequency of bowel movements. Diarrhea is a clinical syndrome of diverse etiology associated with loose or watery stools often with vomiting and fever. Various bacteria, viruses, and parasites cause diarrhea. The most common causes of acute diarrhea are infectious agents [1]. In the Western world, normal fecal weight is less than 200 grams/day with firm to hard consistency of the stools. In India, greater dietary fiber content of the diet increases the fecal mass and its water content. Therefore, it is better to define diarrhea as the condition in which fecal mass and water content are greater than usual. Diarrhea is of two types. One type is called infectious and other is called noninfectious. Bacterium, virus, and parasites cause infectious diseases. Diarrhea affects all age groups but it is most commonly seen in children. Transmission of infection mostly occurs through the fecal-oral pathway. Microscopy and stool cultures are diagnostic investigation for diarrhea. Diarrhea is prevented by precaution such as handwashing. Acute diarrhea

IntechOpen

Cynodon dactylon	Poaceae	Leaves and stems	Antidiarrheal, anti-inflammatory, chemopreventive	[52]
Ziziphus mauritiana	Rhamnaceae	Roots	Antidiarrheal	[53]
Calotropis gigantea	Apocynaceae	Roots, bark, and leaves	Antidiarrheal	[16]
Punica granatum	Lythraceae	Seeds	Antidiarrheal	[36]
Asparagus racemosus	Asparagaceae	Roots	Antidiarrheal	[54]
Xylocarpus moluccensis	Meliaceae	Bark, fruit	Antidiarrheal	[55]
Xylocarpus granatum	Meliaceae	Bark	Antidiarrheal	[56]
Psidium guajava	Myrtaceae	Leaf	Antidiarrheal	[57]
Rhizophora mucronata	Rhizophoraceae	Bark	Antidiarrheal	[58]
Ixora coccinea Linn.	Rubiaceae	Flowers	Antidiarrheal	[59]
Diospyros peregrine	Ebenaceae	Bark	Antidiarrheal	[56]
Moringa oleifera	Moringaceae	Leaf	Antidiarrheal	[60]
Elettaria cardamomum	Zingiberaceae	Fruit	Antidiarrheal	[61]
Mimosa pudica	Fabaceae	Root, leaves	Antidiarrheal, antidepressant, hypolipidemic	[62]
Anthocephalus cadamba	Rubiaceae	Flowering tops	Antidiarrheal	[63]
Alchornea cordifolia	Euphorbiaceae	Leaves	Antidiarrheal	[64]
Nymphaea alba	Nymphaeaceae	Roots, flowers	Antidiarrheal, anxiolytic, anticancer	[65]
Nelumbo nucifera	Nelumbonaceae	Rhizome	Antidiarrheal	[66]
Paederia foetida Linn.	Rubiaceae	Roots, leaves	Antidiarrheal, anti-inflammatory	[67]
Mangifera indica	Anacardiaceae	Seed	Antidiarrheal, immunomodulant, hypoglycemic	[52]
Mezoneuron benthamianum Baill.	Caesalpiniaceae	Leaves	Antidiarrheal, Anti-inflammatory, antipyretic, analgesic	[68]
Piper nigrum L.	Piperaceae	Fruit	Antidiarrheal	[69]
Mimosa pudica	Fabaceae	Leaves	Antidiarrheal	[70]
Cyperus rotundus	Cyperaceae	Roots	Antidiarrheal	[71]

Table 1.
Medicinal plants having antidiarrheal activity.

may also be caused by drugs or toxins. Infectious agents are also responsible for chronic diarrhea. Foods additives, medications, irritable bowel syndrome, malabsorption, and inflammatory bowel diseases are other causes of diarrhea. Diarrhea occurs due to various drugs. Digoxin is usually prescribed for treatment of heart disorders; sometimes diarrhea is seen in the patients taking digoxin. Antibiotics are prescribed for treatment of various ailments including diarrhea, but sometimes it has been observed that diarrhea occurs in the patient taking antibiotics. Diverticulitis is another cause of diarrhea. Infarction of bowel is also responsible for diarrhea [2]. *Salmonella* infection also causes diarrhea that is endemic in Southeast Asia. Other bacterial infections include *Shigella*, *Campylobacter*, *Clostridium difficile*, and *Yersinia*. Toxins of *Staphylococcus aureus*, *Vibrio cholerae*, and *E. coli* are also responsible for diarrhea [3]. Medicinal plants are one of the most popular forms of complementary and alternative medicine. In rural areas, people use medicinal plants as self-medication, and they know medicine for their efficacy in chronic disorders. Therefore, they do not come to doctor for common ailments. Traditional medicine nourishes the body or systems of the body. Medicinal plants have been used since ancient times. This precocious knowledge is transferred from generation to generation. The herbal pharmacopeia has been developed by refining and updating this practice. Gonçalves et al. reported the in vitro anti-rotavirus activity of some medicinal plants used in Brazil against diarrhea [4]. Ojewole et al. reported the antidiarrheal activity of *Psidium guajava* Linn. (Myrtaceae) leaf aqueous extract in rodents [5]. Joshi et al. reported the antidiarrheal activity and chemical profile of *Berberis aristata* [6]. In all cases, the source of diarrhea should be ascertained, and appropriate treatment should then follow. Various modern medicines are originated from plant sources such as aspirin. Plants exert their effects by secondary metabolites present in them. Though a large number of medicinal plants used to treat diarrhea are identified, scientific validation of the medicinal plants of antidiarrheal properties is imperative (**Table 1**). This chapter has shown that multiple plant prescriptions are most commonly used for the management of diarrhea in different systems of medicines.

1.1 Types of diarrhea

1.1.1 Acute diarrhea

Acute diarrhea remains less than 2 weeks. Protozoa, bacteria, virus, food intolerance, and emotional stress cause acute diarrhea [7].

1.1.2 Chronic diarrhea

Chronic diarrhea remains more than 4 weeks.

1.1.2.1 Types of acute diarrhea

Inflammatory diarrhea.
Noninflammatory diarrhea.

1.1.2.1.1 Inflammatory diarrhea

The large intestine is involved in inflammatory diarrhea by invasive parasites or bacteria. Signs and symptoms include fecal urgency, tenesmus, abdominal cramps, fever, small-volume stools, and bloody stool [8].

1.1.2.1.2 Noninflammatory diarrhea

The small intestine is involved in noninflammatory diarrhea. In this type, toxins or viruses affect the small intestine that interferes with water and salt balance. Signs and symptoms include cramps, vomiting, nausea, and large-volume watery diarrhea [9].

1.2 Causes of diarrhea

Causes of diarrhea can be divided into two categories: environmental factors and causative agents.

1.2.1 Environmental factors

Diarrhea is common in bottle-fed children than in breast-fed children. Unhygienic preparations of milk feed, the use of unhygienic bottles, and their contamination by flies and insects may lead to infection of milk, which is an excellent media for the growth and multiplication of organism. On the contrary, breast milk is clean, and it inhibits the growth of organism due to the presence of lactoferrin, lysozymes, leucocytes, macrophages, lactobacillus, and antibodies in it. Infected water and food are also responsible for frequent diarrhea in older children and adults.

1.2.2 Causative agents

Acute diarrhea may be secretory or invasive. Secretory types of diarrhea are caused by bacteria *Vibrio cholerae* and *E. coli*; *Shigella*, *Salmonella*, and *Staphylococcus* may cause invasive diarrhea. Acute diarrhea is also caused by viruses; *Rotavirus* is responsible for 50% of diarrhea in children. Newer viruses like adenoviruses and Norwalk viruses have been found causing diarrhea in children and adults.

1.2.2.1 Cholera

Cholera is a severe acute gastrointestinal infection cause by *Vibrio cholerae*. Transmission is by food or water contaminated by feces from a patient or carrier. Spread may occur from case to case through direct contact with feces. It occurs mostly in hot humid season. *Vibrio cholerae* attach to microvilli of brush border of intestinal epithelium being helped by mucinase. Cholera enterotoxin is released and diarrhea occurs. Stools resemble rice water and contain mucus, epithelial cells, and vibrios. Diagnosis is usually clinical. The presence of rapidly motile vibrios in fresh stool by dark-field illumination is diagnostic. Culture of stool or rectal swabs should be taken [10].

1.2.2.2 Escherichia coli

It consists of two subunits A and B. Subunit B binds to a glycolipid in microvillus membrane. Subunit A enters into cell and inactivates 60S ribosomal subunit. Protein synthesis is stopped and sloughing off of dead cells occurs, and as a result bloody diarrhea occurs [6].

1.2.2.3 Rotavirus

This virus causes typical clinical symptoms of diarrhea preceded or followed by vomiting and fever. It is responsible for 50% diarrheal cases, in children between 6 months and 2 years of age. In developing countries, *Rotavirus* infection is devastating, and lack of treatment leads to high morbidity and mortality [11].

1.2.2.4 Shigella

Shigella dysentery is due to *S. flexneri*, *S. sonnei*, *S. boydii*, and *S. dysenteri*. These four types of serotypes of *Shigella* group produce watery diarrhea and dysentery. *Shigella* dysentery is severe with high mortality. It is a common disease of children below 5 years of age [12].

1.2.2.5 Salmonella

This genus consists of 200 serotypes, which cause diarrhea both in man and animals. *Salmonella* group of organisms causes acute fatal gastroenteritis, enteric fever, bacteremia, and localized infections. These organisms invade the intracellular epithelial cells small intestine. The children are affected more and may continue excrete the organisms up to 2 months after diarrhea has stopped. Indiscriminate use of antibiotics may cause resistance in the organism. Animals are main reservoir, and transmission is passed through food; waterborne and person-to-person transmission is also possible. Enteric fever is a clinical syndrome characterized by gastrointestinal symptoms. Typhoid is the typical form of enteric fever that is caused by *Salmonella typhi*, while a similar less severe illness known as paratyphoid is caused by *Salmonella paratyphi* A, B, or C. Signs and symptoms of typhoid fever include headache, body ache, malaise, sore throat, anorexia, diarrhea, vomiting, stepladder fever, cough, relative bradycardia, palpable spleen, and rose spot rashes [13].

1.2.2.6 *Clostridium perfringens*

It is a spore-bearing bacillus. It causes primarily abdominal cramps and watery diarrhea. Organisms are transmitted through food. In cooked stored food, vegetative cells are destroyed by heat, but spores germinate into vegetative cells on cooling or storing the food [14].

1.2.2.7 *Staphylococcus aureus*

They contain enterotoxins, which are responsible for vomiting and diarrhea. It is a common inhabitant of the human nose, throat, feces, and skin. Foodstuffs like meat and potato stuffs are favorable media for its growth. Enterotoxin being heat stable is not destroyed on heating [15].

1.2.2.8 *Bacillus cereus*

It contaminates soil-grown food and milk. It causes diarrhea and abdominal cramps. It may stimulate staphylococcal food poisoning characterized by nausea and vomiting. Its spores survive at high temperature and boiling and multiply rapidly on cooling and storage.

1.2.2.9 *Entamoeba histolytica*

It invades the large intestine and causes dysentery. Trophozoites containing RBC in stool or cysts are diagnostic. Trophozoites are not infectious but cysts are infectious. Encystment does not occur outside the body. It is passed through uncooked food, water, and from person to person. Cysts of *Entamoeba histolytica* are ingested in water or uncooked food, which has been contaminated by human feces. In the colon, trophozoite forms emerge from the cysts, invading the mucus membrane of the large bowel. The cecum is maximally affected, but any part of the colon may be affected producing flask-shaped ulcers. Sometimes a localized granuloma (ameboma) may present as a palpable mass in the rectum [16].

1.2.2.10 *Giardia lamblia*

It causes watery diarrhea, loose and foul-smelling stools. Abdominal cramps, anorexia, and distension of abdomen are common. Cysts of *Giardia lamblia* are passed through the excreta of man and animals, which infect food. It is also passed through water and person-to-person contact. Infection with *Giardia lamblia* is common in tropical countries. They attach to the mucosa of the duodenum and jejunum and produce inflammation and partial villous atrophy. Signs and symptoms of

Giardia lamblia include loose pale stool, abdominal discomfort, lethargy, nausea, epigastric pain, flatulence, and abdominal distension. For diagnosis, three specimens of stool are collected at 2–3 days interval and examined for cysts within an hour of collections. Duodenal fluid aspiration or jejunal biopsy during endoscopy shows *Giardia lamblia*. For treatment, tinidazole (Fasigyn 500 mg) initially four tabs as a single dose then two tabs daily are given for 5–7 days. Tab. Metronidazole (Flagyl 400 mg) is given three times daily for 5 days [17].

1.3 Levels of dehydration in children with acute diarrhea

1.3.1 Hydration

Sign and symptom of hydration include skin pinch (immediate), drinking (normal), eyes (not sunken), and alertness (normal) [18].

1.3.2 Mild dehydration

Signs and symptoms of mild dehydration include restlessness or irritability, slow skin pinch, drinking eagerly, and sunken eyes [19].

1.3.3 Severe dehydration

Severe dehydration includes very slow skin pinch, drinking poorly or not at all, sunken eyes, and abnormally sleepy or lethargic [20].

1.3.4 Etiology

Etiology of diarrhea includes entero-adhesive *E. coli*, enteropathic *E. coli*, enterotoxigenic *E. coli*, *Shigella*, *Cryptosporidium*, *Giardia lamblia*, *Campylobacter jejuni*, *Salmonella*, disaccharidase deficiency, lactulose, Zollinger-Ellison syndrome (gastrin), phenolphthalein, cascara, senna, partial gastrectomy, blind loop with bacterial overgrowth, lymphoma, adenocarcinoma, radiation enteritis, chronic pancreatitis, pancreatic carcinoma, vagotomy, scleroderma, fistula, small intestinal diverticulitis, allopurinol, celiac disease, tropical sprue, Whipple syndrome, eosinophilic gastroenteritis, Kaposi sarcoma, sarcoidosis, retroperitoneal fibrosis, SSRIs, cholinesterase inhibitors, NSAIDs, proton pump inhibitors, angiotensin II receptor blockers, metformin, ulcerative colitis, Crohn's disease, microscopic colitis, sorbitol, laxative, vipoma, carcinoid, medullary carcinoma of thyroid (calcitonin), and antacids [21].

1.3.5 Host factors

Host factors include malnutrition [22], lactose intolerance, and repeated bouts of diarrhea.

1.3.6 Investigation of diarrhea

Investigation of stool includes stool analysis, stool culture in bloody diarrhea, serum electrolytes, serum urea and creatinine, and sigmoidoscopy if ulcerative colitis is suspected [23].

1.3.7 Principle of treatment

Immune-enhancing drugs should be prescribed to enhance immunity. Diaphoretic drugs are given to control fever. Antimicrobial drugs are prescribed to treat bacterial diarrhea. Anti-inflammatory drugs are given in case of cytotoxins. Gastrointestinal antiseptic herbs can be prescribed. Antiprotozoal herbs are given in case of protozoal infection [24].

1.3.8 Treatment

Soups are advised to patients with diarrhea. Patients are encouraged to take fruit drinks. Caffeine, alcohol, milk products, fats, and high-fiber diets are avoided to rest bowel. Fluids are given at the rate of 5–200 mg/kg/d depending on the hydration state. Intravenous fluids are preferred in patients with severe diarrhea. Normal saline or Ringer's lactate is given to restore water and electrolytes [25].

1.3.9 Oral rehydration therapy

Oral rehydration is given to check or prevent fluid and electrolyte losses and disturbances in all cases of diarrhea of all etiologies. It replaces all fluid and electrolytes in continuing diarrhea. Glucose will provide energy to the body. Glucose by coupling mechanism facilitates absorption of sodium and water. In rural areas where glucose is not available, sucrose of ordinary cane sugar may be used in place of glucose though it is no better than glucose. Sodium and water given orally are poorly absorbed in the small intestine in the absence of glucose. Any safe water can be used for oral rehydration fluid. In case of doubtful hygienic water, it should be boiled and cooled before mixing ingredients in it. In rural areas, the shallow well water are always infected water; therefore boiled and cool water sufficiently treated with bleaching powder should be used. Adequate replacement of potassium loss is particularly important in malnourished children. Sodium bicarbonate rapidly corrects acidosis. Sodium bicarbonate is absorbed during diarrhea. Mild transient alkalosis is of little importance. Its absence from oral rehydration solution shall not lead to bicarbonate bound sodium absorption. This will not only delay the correction of acidosis, but in its absence, acidosis may also become irreversible in many cases.

1.4 Antidiarrheal agents

1.4.1 Anti-motility drugs

Antimuscarinics such as atropine, mepenzolate, propantheline, and dicyclomine are effective in diarrhea. Loperamide is prescribed in diarrhea. Loperamide reduces the intestinal motility. Loperamide only reduces the symptoms of diarrhea. Therefore, cause of diarrhea should be sought [26].

1.4.2 Antibiotic therapy

Metronidazole is prescribed to patients with amebiasis and giardiasis [27]. In acute diarrhea, ciprofloxacin at dose of 200–500 mg twice daily is prescribed for 3 days [28].

1.4.3 Octreotide

This is a somatostatin analogue, which inhibits secretion of local hormones of gastrointestinal tract like gastrin, motilin, VIP, glucagon, and serotonin. Octreotides are prescribed in diarrhea caused by carcinoid tumor, VIPoma, vagotomy, dumping syndrome, short bowel syndrome, and AIDs. Adverse effects include nausea and GIT upsets. Prolonged therapy may cause effects of excessive somatostatin like cholelithiasis [29].

1.4.4 Diphenoxylate

It is available in tablets containing diphenoxylate and atropine. Atropine is added to discourage the addiction liability with diphenoxylate. This combination of diphenoxylate with atropine is known as co-phenotrope [30].

1.4.5 Adsorbents

Kaolin, pectin, chalk, ispaghula, methylcellulose, and sterculia can be used in the treatment of diarrhea, but their effect is weak. Ispaghula, methylcellulose, and sterculia are used in cases of diverticular disease, ileostomy, and colostomy [31].

1.5 Medicinal plants with antidiarrheal and related beneficial properties

1.5.1 Careya arborea Roxb

It belongs to family Lecythidaceae. Leaves and stem are used treat diarrhea. Chemical constituents contain flavonoids, tannins, saponins, and triterpenoids. It is used in bronchitis, cancer, wounds, dysentery, jaundice, diarrhea, boil, ulcer, filaria, swelling, fever, ear pain, skin diseases, stomach diseases, smallpox, body pain, rheumatic pain, eye complaints, asthma, and dental disorders. It is anthelmintic, demulcent, tonic, anticancer, antipyretic, antidiarrheal, antioxidant, antileishmanial, hepatoprotective, and analgesic [11]. The methanol extract of this plant was used for study. Mice were selected for study. Castor oil-induced diarrhea was prevented by the use of *Careya arborea* Roxb. bark. This study indicated that plant has antidiarrheal activity [32].

1.5.2 Berberis lyceum Royle

It belongs to family Berberidaceae. Roots, fruits, leaves, and stem are used to treat diarrhea. Chemical constituents contain palmitine, berberine, iron, zinc, calcium, and vitamin C. It is used in gonorrhea, chronic diarrhea, piles, broken bones, wounds, acute conjunctivitis, jaundice, and diabetes [33]. Pharmacological activities include antioxidant, antidiarrheal, and wound healer [34]. Arshad et al. reported the ethnomedicinal use of this plant in diarrhea [35].

1.5.3 Punica granatum

It belongs to family Lythraceae. Parts used are twig exudates, fruit, flowers, and stem. Chemical constituents contain copper, potassium, phosphorus, sulfur, carotene, vitamin c, fiber, pectin, pelletierine, isopelletierine, iron, calcium, magnesium, calcium, and carbohydrates. It is used in diabetes mellitus, cancer, and cardiovascular disorders. It is antiviral, antibacterial, antidiabetic, chemopreventive, antioxidant, and cardioprotective [36] reported the antidiarrheal activity of *Punica granatum* seed extract in rats. Methanol extract of this plant was used for antidiarrheal activity. Rat models were selected for study. Castor oil-induced diarrhea was prevented by the use of *Punica granatum* seed extract. Charcoal meal test was also performed in rats. Gastrointestinal motility was decreased in rat by the use of extract. This study indicated that plant has antidiarrheal activity.

1.5.4 Trichodesma indicum

It belongs to family Boraginaceae. Parts used are roots. Chemical constituents contain lanast-5-en-3β-D-glucopyranosyl-21 (24)-olide, stigmast-5-en-3β-ol-23-one, n-dotriacont-9-one-13-ene, n-pentacos-9-one, stigmast-5-en-3β-ol-21(24)-olide, n-nonacosanyl palmitate, n-tetradecanyl laurate, and n-decanyl laurate. It is used in dysentery, skin diseases, leprosy, and fever. It is diuretic, antimicrobial, and anti-inflammatory [37]. Antidiarrheal activity of *Trichodesma indicum* was investigated in rat model. Diarrhea was induced by castor oil. Castor oil-induced diarrhea was inhibited by *T. indicum*. This study validated its use in diarrheal disease [37].

1.5.5 *Mentha longifolia*

It belongs to family Lamiaceae. Parts used are dried leaves and young twigs. It is used in diarrhea and dysentery. It is carminative, stimulant, antipyretic, antinociceptive, cytotoxic, insecticidal, calcium channel blocker, and antimicrobial [38]. *M. longifolia* was investigated for its efficacy to treat diarrhea. For this purpose, diarrhea was induced by castor oil. About 100–1000 mg/kg of *M. longifolia* extract exhibited antidiarrheal effect similar to loperamide. High potassium-induced jejunum contraction was inhibited in isolated rabbit jejunum preparations. This indicated its antispasmodic activity through blockage of calcium channels. Calcium concentration curve was shifted rightward with the use of *Mentha longifolia.* This response was similar to verapamil. Inhibition of high K-induced contraction and shifting of calcium concentration curve rightward was also observed by the use of loperamide. Most active fraction was petroleum spirit. This study showed *M. longifolia* antispasmodic and antidiarrheal potential via calcium channel blockade [39].

1.5.5.1 *Acacia nilotica Willd*

It belongs to family Mimosaceae. Parts used are leaves and pods. It is used in diarrhea, dysentery, gonorrhea, diabetes mellitus, sore throat, and cancer [40]. It is anti-plasmodial, chemopreventive, larvicidal, antidiarrheal, hypotensive, and immunomodulant [41]. Antidiarrheal activity of *Acacia nilotica* was investigated. Aqueous, methanol, and petroleum ether extracts were used. Methanol extract exhibited significant antidiarrheal activity. Diarrhea was induced by magnesium sulfate and castor oil. Peristalsis was induced by barium chloride in Swiss albino mice. Antimicrobial activity of *A. nilotica* was investigated against diarrhea-causing organisms. Extract exhibited antidiarrheal potential against magnesium and castor oil-induced diarrhea. Barium chloride peristaltic movements in mice were also reduced by the use of extract. Extract also showed antimicrobial potential against diarrhea-causing organisms. This study validates its use in diarrhea in traditional system of medicine [38].

1.5.5.2 *Alstonia scholaris*

It belongs to family Apocynaceae. Parts used are barks. Chemical constituents contain porphyrin, alstonine, echitamine, picrinine, detamine, and strictamine. This plant has been used in diarrhea, dysentery, and hypertension [42]. It is bronchodilator, antimalarial, spasmolytic, antidiarrheal, anticancer, and neuroleptic. Castor oil-induced diarrhea was prevented by the crude extract of *Alstonia scholaris.* Effective dose of extract was 100–1000 mg/kg. The activity of extract was comparable to standard drug loperamide. This study indicated that plant can be used in diarrhea [39].

1.5.5.3 *Capparis zeylanica L*

It belongs to family Capparaceae. Parts used are flowers and leaves. It is used in diarrhea, cardiovascular disorders, and pyrexia. It is antidiarrheal, antipyretic, antimicrobial, anti-ulcer, and immunostimulant [43]. Methanolic extract of this plant was used for antidiarrheal activity. The activity of plant extract was investigated in castor-induced diarrhea. Mice were selected for study. There was significant reduction in diarrhea in mice. Three level doses (100, 150, and 200 mg/kg) of extract were used for activity. Extract prevented castor oil-induced diarrhea. This activity of plant was comparable to loperamide-treated animals. Intestinal transit was decreased up to 75.97%. This study indicated that plant is effective in diarrhea [44].

1.5.5.4 *Celosia argentea Linn*

It belongs to family Amaranthaceae. Parts used are seeds. It is used in hypertension, inflammation, jaundice, ulcer, skin eruption, and diarrhea. It is antioxidant, antidiarrheal, immunomodulant, antimetastatic, antidiabetic, and wound healer [45]. Alcoholic extract of plant was used for study. Different experimental models were used. Diarrhea was induced by castor oil and PGE (2). Loperamide at dose of 2 mg/kg and atropine at dose of 0.1 mg/kg were used as standard drugs. Two level doses (100 and 200 mg/kg) of extract were used for antidiarrheal activity. Antidiarrheal activity of extract was dose-dependent. This study indicated that plant has antidiarrheal activity [46].

1.5.5.5 *Pentaclethra macrophylla*

It belongs to family Leguminosae. Parts used are leaves and roots. Chemical constituents contain fatty acids, iodine, oil, and carbohydrates. It is used in pruritis, worms, dysentery, cancer, and inflammation. It is antidiarrheal and antidiabetic. Akah et al. reported the antidiarrheal properties of *Pentaclethra macrophylla* leaf extracts. Aqueous and ethanolic extracts of this plant were used for study. Experimental animal models were selected for study. There was significant reduction in fecal output. Extract-treated rats were protected from castor oil-induced diarrhea. Propulsive movements of gastrointestinal contents were significantly decreased in mice. Contractions induced by histamine, nicotine, and acetylcholine were significantly reduced by the use of this extract on isolated tissue preparations. Growth of common pathogenic microorganisms was inhibited. This study showed that plant has antidiarrheal activity [47].

1.5.5.6 *Ficus hispida*

It belongs to family Moraceae. Parts used are leaves. Chemical constituents contain wax, tannin, caoutchouc acid, glucoside, beta-sitosterol, hispidin, bergapten, and psoralen latex. It is used in ulcer, psoriasis, anemia, piles, jaundice, hemorrhage, vitiligo, diarrhea, diabetes, epilepsy, and hepatitis. It is antidiuretic, antibacterial, anti-inflammatory, hypolipidemic, memory enhancer, hepatoprotective, and anticancer [48]. Methanol extract of this plant was used for study. Diarrhea was induced by castor oil. Enteropooling was induced by PGE (2). This study was conducted in rats. Extract prevented diarrhea and enteropooling induced by castor oil and PGE (2). Charcoal meal test was also performed. Gastrointestinal motility was also reduced by the use of this extract. This study indicated that plant has antidiarrheal activity [49].

1.5.5.7 *Terminalia bellirica*

It belongs to family Combretaceae. Parts used are fruit. Chemical constituents contain tannins, beta-sitosterol, chebulagic acid, ethyl gallate, ellagic acid, and gallic acid. It is used in jaundice, tuberculosis, and inflammation. It is antidiarrheal, antioxidant, antispasmodic, hypoglycemic, and bronchodilator [50, 51]. Antidiarrheal activity of plant was investigated. The activity of this plant was also investigated against *E. histolytica*. The activity of plant was investigated against bacteria that cause dysentery and diarrhea. Initially in vitro studies were performed. Furthermore, plant activity was evaluated in clinical trial. Patients having acute and chronic diarrhea and dysentery were selected for study. This study was performed by five medical practitioners. These practitioners were practicing at different clinics. This study was conducted in urban areas of Pune. Clinical trial protocol was given to practitioners. Maximum duration of treatment was 14 days. Bioactive fractions of this plant were used for clinical trial. Tablet was made from bioactive fractions. Tablet was given three times a day at dose of 150 mg. Improvement was observed on second day of treatment. This drug was found effective in diarrhea. Seven patients having amebic dysentery were also recovered attend of treatment. This study indicated that plants are useful for diarrhea and dysentery.

2. Conclusion

This review has revealed that medicinal plants continue to play a vital role in the primary health care of the people. More than half of the people in the world use medicinal plants regularly to treat many ailments, including diarrhea. Hence, further work should be done on the characterization and pharmacological validation of the use of medicinal plants for the treatment of diarrhea. Medicinal plants have potential to treat diarrhea and are prescribed by Unani physician all over the world. Improving hygienic condition prevents diarrhea. Documentation of medicinal plants used to treat diarrhea will help the physician in their practice. There is only description of medicinal plants, but further study should be carried out to find the active constituents responsible for efficacy to treat diarrhea.

Acknowledgements

We acknowledge the Dean Faculty of Medical and Health Sciences for giving permission to conduct research.

Competing interests

Authors declare that there is no conflict of interest.

Funding

There is no funding source.

Ethics approval and consent to participate

Not Applicable.

Consent for publication

There is no identifying information.

Availability of data and material

Data sharing not applicable to this article as no datasets were generated or analyzed during the current study.

Author details

Muhammad Akram[1], Muhammad Daniyal[2*], Aatiqa Ali[3], Iftikhar Ahmed Khan[4], Rida Zainab[1], Khan Usmanghani[5] and Wei Wang[2]

1 Department of Eastern Medicine, Directorate of Medical Sciences, Government College University Faisalabad, Pakistan

2 TCM and Ethnomedicine Innovation and Development International Laboratory, School of Pharmacy, Hunan University of Chinese Medicine, Changsha, China

3 Department of Eastern Medicine, Jinnah University for Women, Karachi, Pakistan

4 Department of Eastern Medicine, Faculty of Medical and Health Sciences, University of Poonch, Rawalakot, Azad Jammu and Kashmir, Pakistan

5 Herbion Pakistan (Pvt.) Ltd., Karachi, Pakistan

*Address all correspondence to: daniyaldani151@yahoo.com

References

[1] Aranda-Michel J, Giannella RA. Acute diarrhea: A practical review. The American Journal of Medicine. 1999;**106**(6):670-676

[2] Daryani NE et al. Colonic diverticular abscess presenting as chronic diarrhea: A case report. Cases Journal. 2009;**2**(1):9389

[3] Nataro JP, Kaper JB. Diarrheagenic *Escherichia coli*. Clinical Microbiology Reviews. 1998;**11**(1):142-201

[4] Gonçalves J et al. In vitro anti-rotavirus activity of some medicinal plants used in Brazil against diarrhea. Journal of Ethnopharmacology. 2005;**99**(3):403-407

[5] Ojewole JA, Awe EO, Chiwororo WD. Antidiarrhoeal activity of *Psidium guajava* Linn.(Myrtaceae) leaf aqueous extract in rodents. Journal of Smooth Muscle Research. 2008;**44**(6):195-207

[6] Jafari A, Aslani M, Bouzari S. *Escherichia coli*: A brief review of diarrheagenic pathotypes and their role in diarrheal diseases in Iran. Iranian Journal of Microbiology. 2012;**4**(3):102

[7] Haberberger R Jr et al. Etiology of acute diarrhea among United States Embassy personnel and dependents in Cairo, Egypt. The American Journal of Tropical Medicine and Hygiene. 1994;**51**(6):870-874

[8] Hodges K, Gill R. Infectious diarrhea: Cellular and molecular mechanisms. Gut Microbes. 2010;**1**(1):4-21

[9] Kovbasnjuk O et al. Human enteroids: Preclinical models of non-inflammatory diarrhea. Stem Cell Research & Therapy. 2013;**4**(1):S3

[10] Moon C et al. Drug-induced secretory diarrhea: A role for CFTR. Pharmacological Research. 2015;**102**:107-112

[11] Gupta PC, Sharma N, Rao CV. Pharmacognostic studies of the leaves and stem of *Careya arborea* Roxb. Asian Pacific Journal of Tropical Biomedicine. 2012;**2**(5):404-408

[12] Zaidi MB, Estrada-García T. Shigella: A highly virulent and elusive pathogen. Current Tropical Medicine Reports. 2014;**1**(2):81-87

[13] Zhang S et al. Molecular pathogenesis of *Salmonella enterica* serotype Typhimurium-induced diarrhea. Infection and Immunity. 2003;**71**(1):1-12

[14] Vaishnavi C, Kaur S. *Clostridium perfringens* enterotoxin in antibiotic-associated diarrhea. Indian Journal of Pathology and Microbiology. 2008;**51**(2):198

[15] Thakkar S, Agrawal R. A case of *Staphylococcus aureus* enterocolitis: A rare entity. Gastroenterology & Hepatology. 2010;**6**(2):115

[16] Haque R et al. Epidemiologic and clinical characteristics of acute diarrhea with emphasis on *Entamoeba histolytica* infections in preschool children in an urban slum of Dhaka, Bangladesh. The American Journal of Tropical Medicine and Hygiene. 2003;**69**(4):398-405

[17] Adam RD. Biology of *Giardia lamblia*. Clinical Microbiology Reviews. 2001;**14**(3):447-475

[18] Lassailly G et al. Bariatric surgery reduces features of nonalcoholic steatohepatitis in morbidly obese patients. Gastroenterology. 2015;**149**(2):379-388

[19] Armstrong LE et al. Mild dehydration affects mood in healthy young women, 2. The Journal of Nutrition. 2011;**142**(2):382-388

[20] Levine AC et al. Ultrasound assessment of severe dehydration in

children with diarrhea and vomiting. Academic Emergency Medicine. 2010;**17**(10):1035-1041

[21] Gasparinho C et al. Etiology of diarrhea in children younger than 5 years attending the Bengo General Hospital in Angola. The Pediatric Infectious Disease Journal. 2016;**35**(2):e28-e34

[22] Ahmed T et al. Management of severe malnutrition and diarrhea. The Indian Journal of Pediatrics. 2001;**68**(1):45-51

[23] Kato J et al. Is sigmoidoscopy sufficient for evaluating inflammatory status of ulcerative colitis patients? Journal of Gastroenterology and Hepatology. 2011;**26**(4):683-687

[24] Mulla WA et al. Evaluation of antidiarrheal and in vitro antiprotozoal activities of extracts of leaves of *Alocasia indica*. Pharmaceutical Biology. 2011;**49**(4):354-361

[25] Davies M, Mayne A. Oral rehydration therapy. Archives of Disease in Childhood. 2001;**84**(3):199

[26] Baker DE. Loperamide: A pharmacological review. Reviews in Gastroenterological Disorders. 2007;**7**:S11-S18

[27] Kimura M, Nakamura T, Nawa Y. Experience with intravenous metronidazole to treat moderate-to-severe amebiasis in Japan. The American Journal of Tropical Medicine and Hygiene. 2007;**77**(2):381-385

[28] Pichler H, Diridl G, Wolf D. Ciprofloxacin in the treatment of acute bacterial diarrhea: A double blind study. Wiesbaden: Vieweg+ Teubner Verlag; Ciprofloxacin. V 1986. pp. 112-114

[29] Bartels MC, Mergenhagen KA. Octreotide for symptomatic treatment of diarrhea due to *Cytomegalovirus colitis*. Annals of Pharmacotherapy. 2011;**45**(1):126-126

[30] Harford WV et al. Acute effect of diphenoxylate with atropine (Lomotil) in patients with chronic diarrhea and fecal incontinence. Gastroenterology. 1980;**78**(3):440-443

[31] Schultz AA et al. Effects of pectin on diarrhea in critically ill tube-fed patients receiving antibiotics. American Journal of Critical Care. 2000;**9**(6):403

[32] Rahman M et al. Antidiarrhoeal activity of the bark extract of *Careya arborea* Roxb. Fitoterapia. 2003;**74**(1-2):116-118

[33] Gulfraz M et al. Comparison of the antidiabetic activity of *Berberis lyceum* root extract and berberine in alloxan-induced diabetic rats. Phytotherapy Research. 2008;**22**(9):1208-1212

[34] Asif A et al. Wound healing activity of root extracts of *Berberis lyceum* Royle in rats. Phytotherapy Research. 2007;**21**(6):589-591

[35] Shedayi AA, Gulshan B. Ethnomedicinal uses of plant resources in Gilgit-Baltistan of Pakistan. Journal of Medicinal Plant Research. 2012;**6**(29):4540-4549

[36] Das AK et al. Studies on antidiarrhoeal activity of *Punica granatum* seed extract in rats. Journal of Ethnopharmacology. 1999;**68**(1-3):205-208

[37] Patwardhan B et al. Clinical evaluation of *Terminalia belerica* in diarrhoea. Ancient Science of Life. 1990;**10**(2):94

[38] Misar A, Bhagat R, Mujumdar A. Antidiarrhoeal activity of *Acacia nilotica* Willd. bark methanol extract. Hindustan Antibiotics Bulletin. 2007;**49**(1-4):14-20

[39] Shah AJ et al. Calcium channel blocking activity of *Mentha longifolia L.* explains its medicinal use in diarrhoea and gut spasm. Phytotherapy Research. 2010;**24**(9):1392-1397

[40] Barapatre A et al. In vitro evaluation of antioxidant and cytotoxic activities of lignin fractions extracted from *Acacia nilotica*. International Journal of Biological Macromolecules. 2016;**86**:443-453

[41] Ahmad S, Mika D. Chemoprotective and immunomodulatory effect of *Acacia nilotica* during cyclophosphamide induced toxicity. Journal of Experimental Therapeutics & Oncology. 2012;**10**(2)

[42] Bello I et al. Mechanisms underlying the antihypertensive effect of *Alstonia scholaris*. Journal of Ethnopharmacology. 2015;**175**:422-431

[43] Ghule B et al. Immunostimulant effects of *Capparis zeylanica* Linn. leaves. Journal of Ethnopharmacology. 2006;**108**(2):311-315

[44] Sharma P et al. Antidiarrhoeal activity of leaf extract of *Celosia Argentea* in experimentally induced diarrhoea in rats. Journal of Advanced Pharmaceutical Technology & Research. 2010;**1**(1):41

[45] Priya KS, Babu M, Wells A. 136 *Celosia argentea* Linn. Leaf Extract Improves Wound Healing in Rat Burn Wound Model. Wound Repair and Regeneration. 2004;**12**(2):A35-A35

[46] Sini KR, Sinha BN, Rajasekaran A. Antidiarrheal activity of *Capparis zeylanica* leaf extracts. Journal of Advanced Pharmaceutical Technology & Research. 2011;**2**(1):39

[47] Akah P, Aguwa C, Agu R. Studies on the antidiarrhoeal properties of *Pentaclethra macrophylla* leaf extracts. Phytotherapy Research: An International Journal Devoted to Pharmacological and Toxicological Evaluation of Natural Product Derivatives. 1999;**13**(4):292-295

[48] Ali M, Chaudhary N. *Ficus hispida* Linn.: A review of its pharmacognostic and ethnomedicinal properties. Pharmacognosy Reviews. 2011;**5**(9):96

[49] Mandal SC, Kumar CA. Studies on anti-diarrhoeal activity of *Ficus hispida.* Leaf extract in rats. Fitoterapia. 2002;**73**(7-8):663-667

[50] Gilani AH et al. Mechanisms underlying the antispasmodic and bronchodilatory properties of *Terminalia bellerica* fruit. Journal of Ethnopharmacology. 2008;**116**(3):528-538

[51] Nampoothiri SV et al. In vitro antioxidant and inhibitory potential of *Terminalia bellerica* and *Emblica officinalis* fruits against LDL oxidation and key enzymes linked to type 2 diabetes. Food and Chemical Toxicology. 2011;**49**(1):125-131

[52] Babu DR et al. Antidiarrheal activity of *Cynodon dactylon*. pers. Pharmacognosy Magazine. 2009;**5**(19):23

[53] Dahiru D, Sini J, John-Africa L. Antidiarrhoeal activity of *Ziziphus mauritiana* root extract in rodents. African Journal of Biotechnology. 2006;(**5**):10

[54] Venkatesan N et al. Anti-diarrhoeal potential of *Asparagus racemosus* wild root extracts in laboratory animals. Journal of Pharmacy & Pharmaceutical Sciences. 2005;**8**(1):39-46

[55] Uddin S et al. Antidiarrhoeal activity of the methanol extract of the barks of *Xylocarpus moluccensis* in castor oil-and magnesium sulphate-induced diarrhoea models in mice. Journal of Ethnopharmacology. 2005;**101**(1-3):139-143

[56] Rouf R et al. Anti-diarrhoeal effects of *Diospyros peregrina* in the castor oil-induced diarrhoea model in mice. ARS Pharmaceutica. 2006;**47**:81-89

[57] Lutterodt GD. Inhibition of Microlax-induced experimental diarrhoea with narcotic-like extracts of *Psidium guajava* leaf in rats. Journal of Ethnopharmacology. 1992;**37**(2):151-157

[58] Rohini R, Das A. Antidiarrheal and anti inflammatory activities of lupeol, quercetin, β-sitosterol, adene-5-en-3-ol and caffeic acid isolated from *Rhizophora mucronata* bark. Der Pharmacia Lettre. 2010;**2**(5):95-101

[59] Maniyar Y, Bhixavatimath P, Agashikar N. Antidiarrheal activity of flowers of *Ixora Coccinea* Linn. in rats. Journal of Ayurveda and Integrative Medicine. 2010;**1**(4):287

[60] Lakshminarayana M et al. Antidiarrhoeal activity of leaf extract of *Moringa oleifera* in experimentally induced diarrhoea in rats. International Journal of Phytomedicine. 2011;**3**(1):68

[61] Rahman T et al. Evaluation of antidiarrhoeal activity of cardamom (*Elettaria cardamomum*) on mice models. Oriental Pharmacy and Experimental Medicine. 2008;**8**:130-134

[62] Balakrishnan N et al. Antidiarrhoeal potential of *Mimosa pudica* root extracts. Indian Journal of Natural Products. 2006;**22**(2):21-23

[63] Alam MA et al. Antidiarrhoeal property of the hydroethanolic extract of the flowering tops of *Anthocephalus cadamba*. Revista Brasileira de Farmacognosia. 2008;**18**(2):155-159

[64] Agbor GA, Léopold T, Jeanne NY. The antidiarrhoeal activity of *Alchornea cordifolia* leaf extract. Phytotherapy Research. 2004;**18**(11):873-876

[65] Bose A, Sahoo M, Ray SD. In vivo evaluation of anti-diarrheal activity of the rhizome of *Nymphaea alba* (Nymphaeaceae). Oriental Pharmacy and Experimental Medicine. 2012;**12**(2):129-134

[66] Mukherjee K et al. Antidiarrhoeal evaluation of *Nelumbo nucifera* rhizome extract. Indian Journal of Pharmacology. 1995;**27**(4):262

[67] Afroz S et al. Antidiarrhoeal activity of the ethanol extract of *Paederia foetida* Linn.(Rubiaceae). Journal of Ethnopharmacology. 2006;**105**(1-2):125-130

[68] Mbagwu H, Adeyemi O. Anti-diarrhoeal activity of the aqueous extract of *Mezoneuron benthamianum* Baill *(Caesalpiniaceae)*. Journal of Ethnopharmacology. 2008;**116**(1):16-20

[69] Shamkuwar PB, Shahi SR, Jadhav ST. Evaluation of antidiarrhoeal effect of Black pepper (*Piper nigrum* L.). Asian Journal of Plant Science and Research. 2012;**2**(1):48-53

[70] Saifiddin Khalid M, Jinesh kumar S, Suresh DK, Kumar R. Evaluation of an anti-diarrhoeal potential of ethanolic extract of *Mimosa pudica* leaves. IJGP. 2011;**5**(1):75-78

[71] Uddin S et al. Antidiarrhoeal activity of *Cyperus rotundus*. Fitoterapia. 2006;**77**(2):134-136

Section 5

Prevention of Acute Diarrhea

Chapter 5

Health Education to Prevent Diarrhea in Preschoolers

Arbianingsih Tiro

Abstract

Preschoolers are the second largest group suffering from diarrhea. Numerous studies have identified poor community hygiene and health practices contributing as causes of diarrhea, making it necessary to teach children healthy behavior for prevention. Healthy behavior can reduce the risk of diarrhea by 36–48%. Unfortunately, health education is commonly given to parents, but it is limited for children. Preschool is a period of transition from parental control to self-control. This period is also the best time to build concepts and ideas with constant reason. Applying an important concept for healthy behavior in this period will help to develop a child's mindset in the future to prevent diarrhea. Health education to prevent diarrhea is pivotal to identify health behavior of preschoolers. When preschoolers' health behavior has been identified, then it can be used to design an effective education model in preventing diarrhea.

Keywords: diarrhea prevention, educational game, healthy behavior, health education, preschoolers

1. Introduction

One of the goals of the Sustainable Development Goals in 2030 is the third goal of reducing child mortality. It is estimated that around 5.9 million children under age five died in 2015 due to preventable diseases [1]. Southeast Asia is the third place for the highest child mortality in the world after sub-Saharan Africa and South Asia. Among ASEAN countries, Indonesia ranks fourth for the highest under-five mortality rate [2]. The most common cause of death of children under five in the world is pneumonia by 18% and diarrhea by 15% [3].

The main factor causing diarrhea is the effect of poor living behavior in the community. The longitudinal study conducted by Santos et al. in preschool children with diarrhea in Brazil found that the duration's determinant of diarrhea was the low ability of the community (low family purchasing power) caused by environmental conditions and children's characteristics and clean behavior [4]. Furthermore, in reducing the incidence of diarrhea, an effective method is selective eating and maintaining personal hygiene [5]. The study conducted by Kariuki et al. in Turkana district, Kenya, found that hygiene and sanitation interventions could reduce the prevalence of diarrhea in children under five from 91.3 to 78.3% [6].

There are several behaviors that can contribute to the incidence of diarrhea, including handwashing with soap, unhealthy snack behavior, and the habit of cutting nails and biting fingers [7, 8]. Those behaviors can contribute to intestinal infections which is one of the causes of diarrhea. Both hands are also the main pathway for the entry of germs into the body because the hands are part of the body most associated with the mouth and nose. The habit of washing hands with soap can reduce the incidence of diarrhea by up to 50% or the same as saving about 1 million children in the world each year [9].

To create healthy behavior, it should be instilled early. Preschool age is an early age for reasoning and constant ideas that are grounded. Planting the concept of healthy behavior at this age will form a healthy lifestyle later on. This preschool period is a transition period from the dominance of parental control to control by the children themselves. In this phase, the children have been able to internalize the standards and values that develop around them, and play is part of the life of preschoolers [10]. The study conducted by Peñalvo et al. stated that health promotion for children aged 3–5 years by integrating behavioral interventions into school curricula in Spain was effective in improving children's healthy behavior [11].

Educating healthy behavior to children in their early life requires appropriate educational strategy. Therefore, things that are needed for that are (1) knowing the behavior of people to prevent health which can be taught to children in school, (2) knowing the health education model that can be applied to children, (3) knowing the effectiveness of the education model that can improve the use of behaviors in diarrhea prevention, and (4) knowing the components of the educational model that must be considered in providing health education.

2. Healthy behavior of diarrhea prevention in preschoolers

Healthy behavior is a person's actions or activities carried out by someone, both directly and indirectly, where habits and practices lead to ways to maintain, restore, and improve their health and prevent the risk of disease [12, 13]. Healthy behavior is important to be taught early because this will form a healthy lifestyle in the future. Children who understand healthy behavior will be familiar and not easily lost at the next stage of development. Children will learn healthy behaviors from what they see, hear, and experience. For children in this age group, the most pleasant and effective method is playing, which is a way for children to understand, adjust, and develop life experiences [14].

There are eight indicators of healthy and clean life behavior for early childhood (refer to the Ministry of Health). Eight school healthy and clean life behavior indicators, which can be applied to early childhood, are washing hands with running water and using soap, consuming healthy snacks in the school canteen, using clean and healthy latrines, eradicating mosquito larvae, not smoking in schools, exercising regularly, measuring weight and height each month, and disposing of garbage in its place [15]. Briefly, there are five healthy behaviors in preschoolers that can be intervened [13, 16]:

- Washing hands with running water and using soap: Germs and viruses can survive up to 2 hours on the surface of the skin, tables, door handles, toys, and so on. Hand hygiene that is not properly maintained can cause diseases such as diarrhea, cough, runny nose, and fever. It is crucial to know how to wash hands well and encourage children to wash their hands before eating, after playing, after going to the toilet, and after traveling.

- Consuming nutritious foods: It is pivotal to advice children to be careful in eating snacks and food/drinks. Parents should serve children balanced nutritious foods, including staple foods (rice, noodles, and rice noodles), side dishes (meat, fish, chicken, tofu, and *tempe*), vegetables, and fruit every day. Making eating activities is a fun time. Do not force children to eat because the most important thing for children is not the quantity of food but the quality of what they eat.

- Maintaining environmental cleanliness: Some activities that children can perform are disposing garbage in its place, putting shoes in place, putting dirty eating utensils in place, using footwear when being outside of the house, covering the mouth when coughing and sneezing, keeping away from cigarette smoke, kitchen smoke, smoke burning garbage, and motor vehicle fumes, cleaning toys regularly, and defecating and urinating in the toilet.

- Using clean water and clean latrines for daily needs: It is important to teach children to defecate in the toilet. Encourage children to use clean water for bathing twice a day, shampooing every other day, brushing their teeth at least twice a day, cleaning their ears every time they shower, and washing their feet after each trip and each time going up to bed.

- Do not smoke and do physical activities: Teach children about the dangers of smoking for health. Regular physical activity is important for improving well-being and maintaining physical fitness [17].

Healthy behavior varies due to several factors, including (1) access to healthcare facilities, (2) attitudes toward health workers, (3) perceptions of disease threats, (4) knowledge of diseases, (5) characteristics of social networks, and (6) demographic factors. The second to fifth factors are part of cognitive factors (beliefs, attitudes, and knowledge). Cognitive factors are determinants of the most important intrinsic factors for changing behavior [12].

In short, the important healthy behaviors that need to be taught to preschoolers are handwashing practices, clean eating practices, and eating balanced nutrition.

2.1 Handwashing practice

Handwashing with soap is one of the clean and healthy behaviors. Nowadays, the behavior of washing hands with soap has become a worldwide concern because the problem of lack of practice of handwashing behavior does not only occur in developing countries but also in developed countries. Thereby, the United Nations (UN) general meeting stipulated the Global Handwashing Day on October 15, 2008. This is a manifestation of the need to improve the practice of personal hygiene and sanitation throughout the world. The Global Handwashing Day which is celebrated by many countries in the world is an effort to improve handwashing with soap culture globally, so that the spread of diseases caused by the environment and human behavior such as diarrheal diseases can be reduced [18]. The behavior of handwashing with soap can reduce gastrointestinal disease by 31% and respiratory tract disease by 21%. Washing hands using non-antibacterial soap shows greater benefits than antibacterial soap [19].

Washing hands with soap is an effort to prevent disease. This is done because hands often become agents that carry germs and cause pathogens to move from one person to another, either by direct contact or indirect contact (using other surfaces such as towels and glasses). Hands that come in direct contact with human and animal feces or other body fluids (such as snot) and contaminated food/drinks when not washed with soap can move bacteria, viruses, and parasites to other people who are not aware that they are being infected [1].

Handwashing with soap should be done at five important times: (1) before eating, (2) after defecation, (3) before holding the baby, (4) after changing diapers or cleaning up a child who has used the toilet, and (5) before preparing food. Washing hands using soap and running water can break the germ chain attached to the fingers. Communities including children often ignore handwashing using soap with running water because of a lack of understanding of health [17].

Factors that influence handwashing behavior: (1) environment (parents, caregivers, teachers, friends, and customs); (2) body image showing the importance of maintaining cleanliness for the individual; (3) knowledge about the importance of cleanliness and motivation of individuals in the care of personal hygiene; (4) culture, belief, and individual personal values for personal hygiene care; and (5) socioeconomic status [20].

According to the WHO, there are 10 steps in washing hands with soap and water: (1) wet hands with water; (2) apply hand soap; (3) flatten soap with both hands until the palms are exposed to soap; (4) rub the back of the right hand with the left hand until between the fingers then alternately the left hand; (5) put the palms together with the fingers crossed between fingers; (6) place the back of the finger on the other palm with fingers interlocking; (7) rub the thumb by holding the left thumb with the right hand and then rotating the opposite; (8) rub the fingers of the right hand on the left hand to clean the nails of the right hand, and vice versa; (9) rinse with running water; and (10) use a dry and clean towel or disposable tissue to dry your hands (**Figure 1**) [22].

2.2 Clean eating practices

One factor that causes diarrhea in children is consuming unhealthy foods. Elementary school children like to eat ice and cakes where many food processing does not meet hygiene standards. Some of them are preparation and storage of food ingredients, cross-contamination from raw materials to cooked foods, less clean cooking utensils, and ingredients that use coloring agents, preservatives, or artificial sweeteners. This can cause digestive problems in children causing diarrhea [23].

The results of the study conducted by Pradipta et al. found that there was a relationship between hygienic snacking habits and the incidence of diarrhea where children who had more unhygienic snacking habits experienced diarrhea. Unhealthy snacks are snacks that contain artificial food colors and food that is infested with flies or other insects. In addition to food sanitation, sanitation of tableware also needs attention [24]. It is important to teach children that if they are eating and utensils fall on the floor, they should be washed before using it again, and if the food falls on the floor, it should not be eaten [25].

2.3 Eating a balanced diet

Balanced nutrition is food consumed by individuals in 1 day that is diverse and contains energy, building materials, and regulating substances according to their body needs [26]. Nutritional needs are a very crucial requirement in helping the process of growth and development in children. Malnutrition in children causes children to be susceptible to disease. Poor nutritional status causes children to experience diarrhea [27].

The consumption pattern of balanced nutrition quality food requires the need for food diversification in the daily menu. This requires the availability of energy sources (carbohydrates and fats), sources of building materials (proteins), and sources of regulatory substances (vitamins and minerals). Diverse food is very important because there is no one type of food that can provide nutrition for a person in full [28].

DOI: http://dx.doi.org/10.5772/intechopen.86414

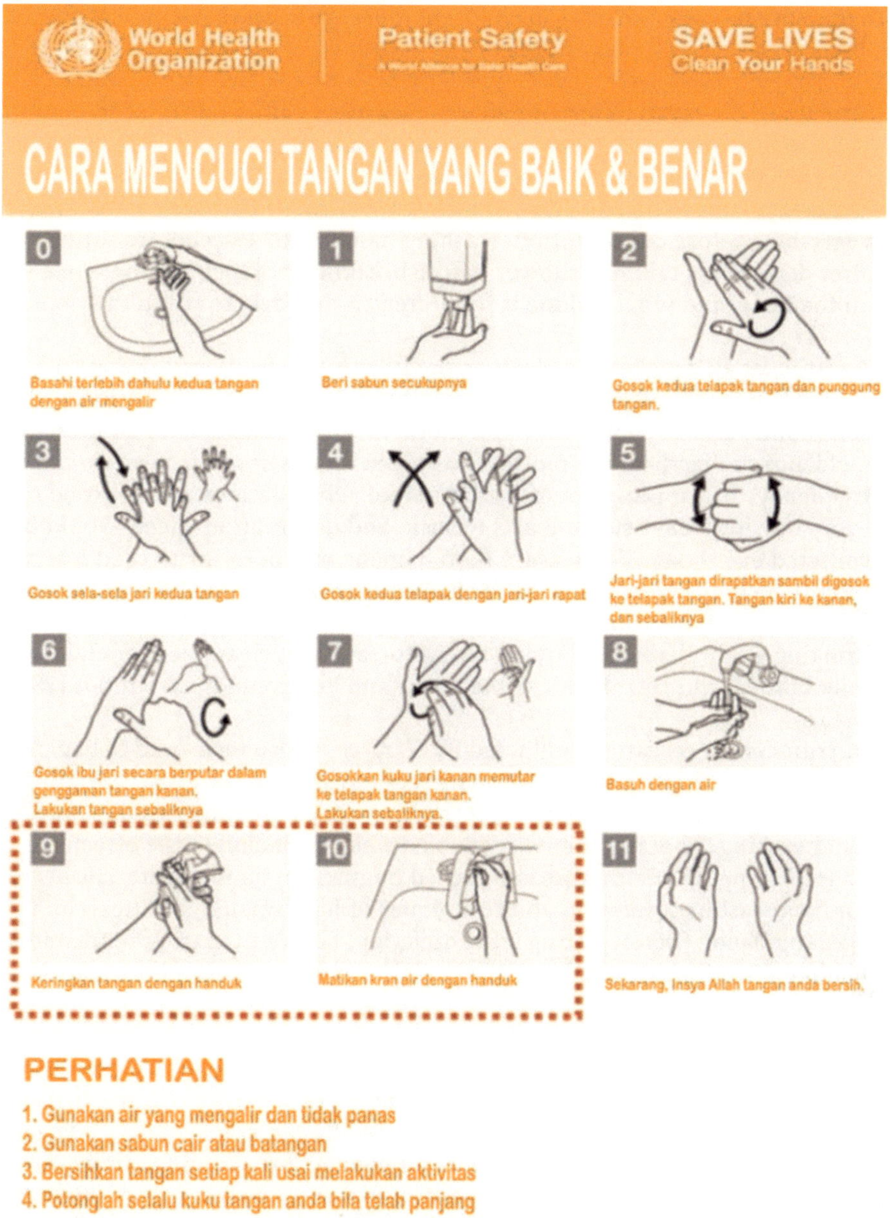

Figure 1.
How to wash hands properly and correctly [22].

The National Agency of Drug and Food Control of Republic of Indonesia (NADFC) 2013 exemplifies the composition of balanced nutrition in school children consisting of:

- Carbohydrates: rice, noodles, corn, bread, sweet potatoes, cassava
- Protein: meat, fish, chicken, tempe/tofu, eggs, milk
- Vegetables: spinach, mustard, tomatoes, carrots, water spinach
- Fruit: banana, papaya, pineapple, watermelon, apples

To measure healthy behavior in children, there are several instruments that have been used by several previous studies:

- Structured observation instruments to measure healthy behavior in children and their caregivers developed by Strina et al. which consisted of 23 items of hygienic and unhygienic behavior related to the incidence of diarrhea [12]. Generally, the observed items included the source of drinking water, washing vegetables before consumption, washing hands with soap before eating and after defecation, taking a shower before breakfast or lunch, eating while sitting on the floor, and what is done if food/utensils and drinks fall to the floor.

- Agustina et al. developed a clean eating practice instrument for diarrhea children in Indonesia based on the results of a survey and discussion with community health center staff and mothers with preschoolers. To measure the incidence of diarrhea, the mother was given an observation sheet on the time, frequency, and appearance of a child's stool. Observations were carried out every day for 7 days starting at 8 o'clock, and observation sheets would be collected every day. To measure food hygiene practices, structured interviews refer to 36 items which include the behavior of mother and child handwashing, food preparation, cleaning of kitchen equipment, sources and safety of drinking water, habits of buying ready-to-eat food, cleanliness of children's milk bottles, and cleanliness of the house and environment around it [29].

- Instruments in research conducted by Garg et al. also measured behavior in children related to handwashing. The semi-structured questionnaire filled by children was developed to find out the knowledge and practice of handwashing. The questionnaire items developed included the effects of handwashing on health, diseases caused by unclean hands, materials needed for handwashing, duration and techniques of handwashing, critical time for washing hands (before eating, after toileting, before preparing food, and after holding dirty items), handwashing practices, and sources of information.

Moreover, Kim et al. developed behavioral instruments to identify handwashing behavior, the stages of behavior change, self-efficacy, positive or negative attitudes, and a food safety knowledge [16]. The instrument consists of five parts that measure [1]: proper handwashing behavior, measured by the Likert scale 1 = never and 5 = always [2]; identify the stages of behavior change, measured by giving three options: do not consider handwashing behavior important, consider handwashing behavior important even though they have not practiced it well, and realize the importance of handwashing behavior and will apply it within the next 6 months [3]; knowing self-efficacy, measured using the item "I can wash my hands after I get out of the bathroom despite being in a hurry" with scoring 1 = completely unsure and 5 = very confident [4]; knowing positive or negative attitudes; and a food safety knowledge questionnaire consisting of 10 items [16].

3. Health promotion model to change health behavior in preschoolers

Health programs for preschool children generally focus on developing children's sense of responsibility for their health and safety. The main thing for this condition is an increase in knowledge about health habits. Therefore, activities provided for preschool children in teaching basic habits about hygiene and more specifically help them (a) realize the importance of health, nutrition, personal hygiene, and exercise to maintain health, (b) learn basic rules of hygiene (handwashing, brushing teeth, etc.), (c) distinguish between substances and healthy and hazardous foods, and (d) learn about the role of several health services and be informed about the risks of disasters that can occur such as fires, earthquakes, floods, etc. and learn how to protect themselves.

There are several health promotion models that can change healthy behavior in children as follows.

3.1 Educational game

An educational game is very interesting to develop. There are several advantages of educational game compared to conventional education methods. One of the main benefits of the educational game is the visualization of real problems. The Massachusetts Institute of Technology (MIT) succeeded in proving that games are very useful for improving the logic and understanding of players about a problem through a game project called Scratch. Based on the results of previous studies, there is no doubt that educational game can support the educational process [30, 31]. Educational games excel in several aspects when compared to conventional learning methods. One significant advantage is the existence of animation that can improve memory so that children can store subject matter in a longer time than conventional teaching methods [32]. Simulation-based educational games are designed to simulate existing problems so that essences or knowledge can be used to solve these problems. Simulation games can be used as one of the educational media that can be learned and done individually. Based on the patterns possessed by the game, players are required to learn so that they can solve existing problems. The status of the game, instructions, and tools provided by the game will actively guide players to explore information so that it can enrich their knowledge and strategies while playing.

3.2 Sociodrama

Health education that incorporates therapeutic sociodramatic games can help school-age children to change their behavior. School-age children are in the development with concrete stages in which they can reflect on events and actions that they see in real terms. The sociodramatic play reflects real events, so it can motivate children to act according to what they experience during role-playing. For example, a child who plays the role of a patient suffering from diarrhea will be encouraged to believe that it is not optimal to be infected with the disease; thus it motivates the child to develop preventative behavioral diarrhea. Peers play an important role in developing health and hygiene behavior, which is why researchers have chosen them as role partners, making this relationship in an effort to better describe diarrhea prevention behaviors. Therefore, a sociodramatic therapeutic game is expected to improve the prevention of diarrhea among school-age children.

Sociodramatic games improve diarrhea prevention behavior in school children. This interactive health education method meets the needs and developmental stages of school-age children. Therapeutic sociodramatic games involve the concept of learning while working and by directly practicing healthy behavior. It can accelerate the process of behavior change, which will help in strong memorization by school-age children. Therapeutic sociodramatic games have become a variety of nursing interventions in the form of interesting games among school-age children. Therapeutic sociodramatic games can also be integrated into school subject curricula, such as arts and culture, physical education, and cocurricular activities as programs to promote preventive behavior by the health movement in schools.

3.3 Educational video

An educational video is one of the health promotion methods for Preschoolers. This is effective because the information received or stimuli that enter through the five senses, visually through the eyes and hearing through the ears, will be recorded by sensory memory. If the information or stimuli are not taken care of, they will be immediately forgotten, but if you pay attention, the information will be transferred to the short-term memory system. After being in the short-term memory system, the information is transferred again with the repetition process to the long-term memory system to be stored [33].

3.4 Singing

The most effective method in changing behavior, from behavior that is detrimental to health toward behavior that benefits health, is through health education. Health education can be done using various methods, one of which is the singing method. The singing method is very appropriate given to preschoolers because it is a fun method that makes children more active and creative, and the lessons are given more effective for children [34].

From some of the studies above, an effective promotion model used in children is through playing activities that include educational activities, videos, role play and songs. Referring to these health promotion models that are declared effective, they can actually be combined in one game model. Games can also help children to practice making the same decisions with real life without risk [35].

In the digital era, gadgets are the main requirement. It also appears that the type of game that children love today is playing games. Nowadays, the use of video games in children is increasing. In the United States, boys and girls have an average of 5.5 hours/week playing games [36]. Children aged 2–7 years in the Netherlands spend an average of 3–5 hours/week playing games, and children aged 8–9 years spend an average of 9 hours/week playing games [37]. Thereby, games are a great potential to be used as an educational medium for preschoolers.

4. The effectiveness of educational games on improving children's healthy behavior

Intervention using games to change behavior is now one of the ways in health promotion in groups of children. Some studies depict that participants show positive behavioral changes after they are given a game playing intervention. In-game stories allow players to imitate, gain identified experiences from others, and learn about the moral contained in the story. A comprehensive model for learning to change behavior in video games is based on social cognitive theory and elaboration likelihood models that include the stages of attention, retention, production, and motivation. Baranowski et al. propose a conceptual model of variables that mediate behavior change. This concept model is based on components of four theories, namely, the theory of self-determination, transportation, elaboration probability, and social cognitive [38].

The theory of self-determination states that motivation initiates changes in a person's behavior primarily intrinsic motivation. Video games can motivate children by first motivating children to start playing, keep playing, and change behavior. Transportation theory states that to change behavior, someone must be able to dissolve in the story so that it is easy to influence through the message in the story.

Elaboration likelihood model states that getting and maintaining someone's attention is the first step to provide information to someone to change behavior. The social cognitive theory states that changes in a person's behavior are a function of increasing one's skills and self-efficacy to perform new behaviors [38] (**Figure 2**). The following is a conceptual model framework for how video games affect behavior change:

Stories in a game are made so that players can be dissolved in the story and focus on characters with the expected behavior model. Behavior simulation can be done by providing a virtual environment so that children are familiar with behavioral skills. Behavioral procedures can be introduced by giving an opportunity to players to try behavior changes through their character in the game. Although various studies related to video games have measured outcome such as knowledge to complex behavioral changes, it is not possible to know changes in attributes of specific components of the game due to the complexity of the game itself [39]:

- Factors that encourage learning or the implementation of behavior that is influenced by media [14].
- Age. Young children focus on behavior and not on motivation or effect. They see alternatives as concrete, and they remember things in the program.
- Identifying characters or situations. Children will more often imitate the behavior of others and the same situation with people and situations in their own lives.
- Award and punishment syndromes. Children will imitate the behavior they see as valued or not punished if the behavior is desired. They tend to rarely repeat an action they see being punished, and their attention is immediately attracted when they see an action that they know must be punished but apparently not punished.
- Opportunity to reproduce behavior. Children will imitate behavior when given the right environment or if violence seems to be an acceptable solution. When children see the situation on television, they will use this information if they face a similar situation that requires resolution.

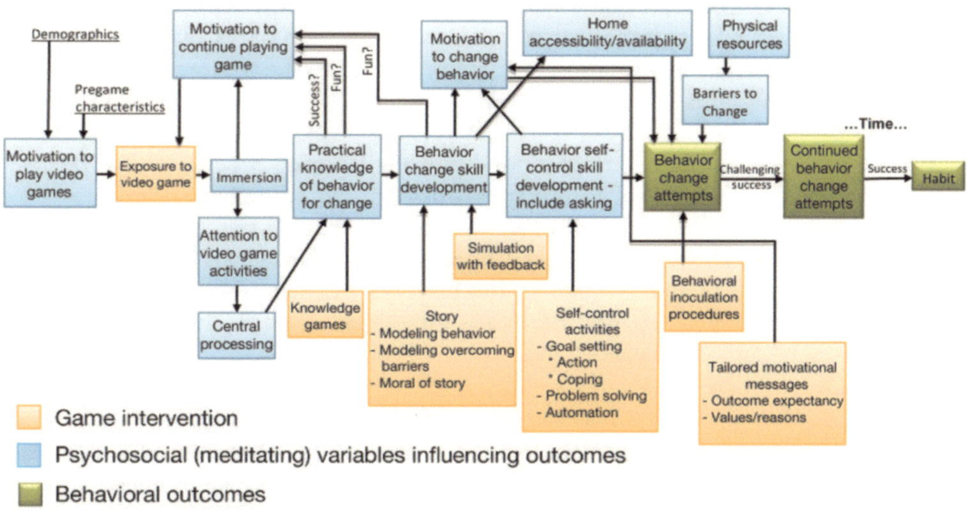

Figure 2.
The conceptual framework of video games influences behavior change.

- Motivation to reproduce behavior. Children will imitate behavior when given the right payment: expect appreciation or no punishment. Some children have self-control, while the other children do not have it.

- The game becomes one of the effective methods of learning activities in children. This was stated by Teed in a study of game-based learning (GBL) [40]. Games are effective in elevating learning activities because games are able to motivate students to learn. The process of learning through games begins with children's interest in the game where the game is seen as fun and capable of drowning them in the material so that they learn more effectively. Furthermore, learning through games is able to encourage students to learn from their mistakes in the game so as to make children learn from their decision-making mistakes in playing. These reasons prove that play is an appropriate method that can be used to improve children's knowledge. The game has great potential to be used as a method of increasing knowledge early so that it is expected to have an effect on achieving a behavior that supports the creation of improved health status and is more permanent for children in the future.

- In addition to knowledge, the core concept that promotes increased healthy behavior through gameplay is self-efficacy.

- Mikropoulos and Natsis state that self-efficacy affects students' choices in learning. Through self-efficacy, students can be more challenged in learning and have the ability to survive to learn even in difficult conditions [21, 22]. Ketelhut who observed 7-year-olds who played virtual games about the environment shows that students who have high self-efficacy also display better behavior [41].

- In playing games, players will be brought in a narrative story game which is a flow of information that delivers games to a concept of an educational game. According to the narrative-centered learning theory developed by Gerrigs (1993), there are two cognitive processes of a comprehensive narrative. Firstly, the readers will be taken to a place and time where they will feel like they are in the real world. Secondly, they will play their own stories, draw conclusions, and gain emotional experiences from interactions with narratives [23]. The game also provides information that is narrative, so students learn from the narrative experiences that they obtain.

- Self-efficacy is an important component of the learning process. Self-efficacy affects understanding and appearance, an adaptation of behavior, and conditions to be achieved. Self-efficacy refers to the self-perception of a person's skills and abilities to do action well. Self-efficacy is formed through change intolerance at each stage of the behavior change process. Hence, self-efficacy is a pivotal precondition that is important to be maximized in achieving behavior change.

- Feist and Gregory perceive that there are four factors that influence self-efficacy, namely, past experience of the success of carrying out these actions, the influence of social modeling seen from role models, social persuasion, and physical and emotional status. After the intervention, the children are no longer given any intervention and are merely observed. This condition will show how much behavior they have learnt is internalized into their daily life.

Preschool children's self-efficacy assessment in this study based on statement aspects and appearance aspects. Many aspects that have decreased are aspects of appearance [26].

- The majority of educational games have an impact on children's knowledge, attitudes, and motivations [27]. Educational games have a primary target for behavioral mediators such as self-efficacy. This change in the behavior mediator is expected to produce the expected behavior. The selection of the target mediator is based on a theoretical basis that is used as a source in developing strategies to change behavior [39].

- The theory of Fisch's capacity model in Lavigne's paper states that the success of transferring learning outcomes depends on the child's ability to produce concepts that represent the appearance of television and the ability to identify similar contexts in daily life [28]. In Nola J. Pender's health promotion model theory, practice is the expected result of a series of behavioral change processes. Therefore, altering practices is the last component to be achieved in a health promotion intervention through educational games for preschoolers.

5. The components of game favored by children

The attractive components of game as a medium of education for children need to be known. This is the key in ensuring the effectiveness of a game as an educational medium. The result of the study in investigating game components favored by children conducted by the author can be considered in designing the game as the educational media for the characteristics of the main character, the model of the game presented, and the color that dominates the game.

The characteristics of the main character that children enjoy in a game are moving creatures or object, consisting of evolutionary and an attractive appearance. The main character is one of the main things that attracts kids to play a game. If the main character is interesting, the children will try to play the game. This is important in the development of educational games because the attraction of children to play games is a step forward in providing educational information [29]. One of the characters of the game that is also appealing and is loved by preschoolers is a funny and cheerful character [42]. Preschoolers aged 3–5 years old have imaginative playing characteristics which are both fantasy and informal. The imagination provides an opportunity for players to experience decision-making of problem resolution in risk-free conditions [35]. This will create a pleasant learning environment for children as well as stimulate improvement in mindset.

In developing the method for preschoolers, it must take into account four things that are clear and consistent instruction, challenging learning environment, having a choice in controlling the game, and having an attractive appearance. An attractive display includes images of background, image descriptions, and sound that are appropriate with children. An appealing appearance of the game will increase the interest of children in the learning process. Therefore, it will stimulate cognitive cognition of children in the learning process.

The characteristics of the game that are loved by children are varied such as giving prizes and having varied games. Preschool age is the best age to learn quick. Children have great curiosity and want to know things about work [43]. Preschoolers also have psychographic characteristics that are like being active, high curiosity, happy to be involved with something new, and having high creativity [44]. Schoolchildren enjoy imitative, imaginative, and dramatic games where in the game can give them the right condition to express themselves. Preschoolers are generally given cognitive game [42]. In educating preschoolers, it needs components: audiovisual, interaction, termination, and positive reinforcement to result positive learning process.

Positive reinforcement is pivotal in developing educational game to increase children's motivation particularly intrinsic motivation. This may motivate children to play and learn something so as to they can feel the story of the game. The game players may obtain active learning experience, so it may elevate children's ability in analyzing, synthesizing, and evaluating [35].

The primary colors used are red, yellow, and blue and the secondary colors are green, orange, purple, and pink. Children are fonder of learning through visually interesting, colorful, and interactive objects than just textbook and oral learning. Video games with color, sound, and attractive appearance significantly increase children's interest in learning. This will lead to dissolution in the education message delivered through the game. All the interests are increasingly becoming more important for learning, so that this will increase the motivation of children in learning.

6. Conclusion

Health education to prevent diarrhea is important to identify health behavior of preschoolers. When preschoolers' health behavior has been identified, then it can be used to determine an effective education media in preventing diarrhea. The basic healthy behaviors to be taught to children are washing hands using soap in critical time, healthy eating behavior, and eating balanced nutrition. The effective educational medium to teach healthy behavior in preschool children is game. The components of a game favored by children are the main character, the model, and dominant color of the game.

Acknowledgements

I would like to thank A. Adriana Amal and Fitriani for their assistance in translation in order to write this chapter. I would also like to thank all authors whose works I cited in this work for their valuable contribution to knowledge.

Conflict of interest

The author declares no conflict of interest.

Author details

Arbianingsih Tiro
Alauddin State Islamic University, Makassar, Indonesia

*Address all correspondence to: arbianingsih.tiro@uin-alauddin.ac.id

References

[1] WHO. The Sustainable Development Goals Report 2017 [Internet]. Washington, USA; 2017. Available from: https://www.paho.org/hq/index.php?option=com_docman&view=download&category_slug=160-en-9007&alias=40341-ce160-14-e-341&Itemid=270&lang=en

[2] Ministry of Health. Indonesia Health Profile (in Indonesian) [Internet]. 2014. pp. 1-382. Available from: http://www.depkes.go.id/resources/download/pusdatin/profil-kesehatan-indonesia/profil-kesehatan-indonesia-2012.pdf

[3] Faijer DJ, Bay G, Miller T. UNICEF. Level and Trends in Child Mortality; 2011

[4] Santos CAST, Strina A, Amorim LD, Genser BB, Assis AMO, Prado MS, et al. Individual and contextual determinants of the duration of diarrheal episodes in preschool children: A longitudinal study in an urban setting. Epidemiology Infection. 2012;**140**(4):689-696

[5] Liyold R, Bennnett C. Travellers' diarrhea: Causes, prevention and treatment. Nursing Standard. 2012;**26**(40):51-56. DOI: 10.7748/ns2012.06.26.40.51.c9137

[6] Kariuki JG, Magambo KJ, Njeruh MF, Muchiri EM, Nzioka S. Effects of hygiene and sanitation interventions on reducing diarrhoea prevalence among children in resource constrained communities: Case study of Turkana District, Kenya. Journal of Community Health. 2012;**37**(6):1178-1184. Available from: https://www.ncbi.nlm.nih.gov/pubmed/22477669

[7] Rosidi A, Handarsari E, Mahmudah M. The relationship of handwashing habit and food sanitation with diarrhea incidence in children of podo 2 elementary school, Kedungwuni District, Pekalongan regency (in Indonesian). Journal Kesehatan Masyarakat Indonesia. 2012;**6**:76-84

[8] Rompas MJ, Tuda J, Ponidjan T. The relationship of handwashing with soap with the incidence of diarrhea in children (in Indonesian). Journal Keperawata. 2013;**1**:1-8

[9] Team GHD. Planner 's Guide

[10] Hockenberry MJ, Wilson D. Wong's Essentials of Pediatric Nursing. 8th ed. Canada: Mosby Elsevier; 2009

[11] Peñalvo JL, Santos-Beneit G, Sotos-Prieto M, Martínez R, Rodríguez C, Franco M, et al. A cluster randomized trial to evaluate the efficacy of a school-based behavioral intervention for health promotion among children aged 3 to 5. BMC Public Health. 2013;**13**(1):1-6

[12] Strina A, Cairncross S, Barreto ML, Larrea C, Prado M. Childhood diarrhea and observed hygiene behavior in Salvador, Brazil. American Journal of Epidemiology. 2003;**157**(11):1032-1038

[13] Agustina R, Sari TP, Satroamidjojo S, Bovee-oudenhoven IMJ, Feskens EJM, Kok FJ. Association of food-hygiene practices and diarrhea prevalence among Indonesian young children from low socioeconomic urban areas. BMC Public Health. 2013;**13**:977

[14] Widjaja M. Mastering Diarrhea and Poisoning in Toddlers (In Indonesian). Jakarta: Kawan Pustaka; 2000

[15] Garg A, Taneja DK, Badhan SK, Ingle GK. Impact of a school-based hand washing promotion program on knowledge and hand washing behavior of girl students in a middle school of Delhi. The Lancet. 2013;**57**(2):57-60

[16] Kim EJ, Pai AJ, Kang N, Kim WK, Kim YS, Moon H. The effects of food safety education on adolescents' hand

hygiene behavior: An analysis of stages of change. KoreaMed Synapse. 2012; **6**(2):169-174

[17] Thompson D, Baranowskia T, Cullen K, Watson K, Liu Y, Canada A, et al. Design of video games for children's diet and physical activity behavior change. International Journal of Computer Science in Sport. 2014; **9**(2):3-17

[18] Ministry of Health. Handbook for Eradicating Diarrhea (in Indonesia). Jakarta: Ditjen PPM & PL; 2009

[19] Aiello AE, Coulborn RM, Perez V, Larson EL. Effect of hand hygiene on infectious disease risk in the community setting: A meta-analysis. American Journal of Public Health. 2011;**98**(8): 1372-1381

[20] Eko L. The Relationship between the Habit of Washing Hands of Pre-School Children and the Incidence of Diarrhea in the Working Area of the Surakarta Public Health Center (in Indonesian). Surakarta: Universitas Muhammadiyah; 2012

[21] Mikropoulos TA, Natsis A. Educational virtual environments: A ten-year review of empirical research (1999–2009). Computers in Education. 2011;**56**(3):769-780. Available from: http://dx.doi.org/10.1016/j.compedu.2010.10.020

[22] WHO. Guidelines on Hand Hygiene in Health Care First Global Patient Safety Challenge. Switzerland: WHO Press; 2009

[23] Meluso A, Zheng M, Spires HA, Lester J. Enhancing 5th graders' science content knowledge and self-efficacy through game-based learning. Computers in Education. 2012;**59**(2): 497-504

[24] Khomsan A. Food and Nutrition for Health (in Indonesian). Jakarta: PT Raja Grafindo Persada; 2004

[25] Pradipta HA, Noor S. The relationship of snacking behavior with the diarrhea incidence in elementary school children: In Cempaka district, Banjarbaru (in Indonesian). Berkala Kedokteran. 3 June 2016;**9**(1): 93-100

[26] Feist J, Gregory JF. Theories of Personality. 7th ed. Boston: McGraw-Hill Higher Education; 2009

[27] Connolly TM, Boyle EA, Arthur EM, James T. A systematic literature review of empirical evidence on computer games and serious games. Computers in Education. 2012;**59**(2):661-686

[28] Lavigne H. The Priming Effects of Video Viewing on Preschoolers Play Behavior. Massacchusetts: University of Massachusetts; 2012

[29] Baranowski T, Buday R, Thompson DI, Baranowski J. Playing for real: Video games and stories for health-related behavior change. Medicine (Baltimore). 2009;**34**(1):74-82

[30] Clark RE. Evaluating the Learning and Motivation Effects of Serious Games. Rosier School of Education Center for Creative Technologies; 2006. Available from: http://projects.ict.usc.edu/itgs/talks/Clark_Serious.Games Evaluation.ppt

[31] Clark RE, Choi S. Five design principles for experiments on the effects of animated pedagogical agents. Journal of Educational Computing Research. 2005;**32**(3):209-225

[32] Clark D. Games and e-learning. Sunderland: Caspian Learning; 2006

[33] Bhinnety M. Structure and process of memory. Buletin Psikologi. 2008;**16** (2). DOI: https://doi.org/10.22146/bpsi.7375

[34] Listyowati. The Use of German Singing Method in German Language

Learning in Class X3 High School Laboratory of Universitas Negeri Malang (in Indonesian)

[35] Akl EA, Kairouz VF, Sackett KM, Erdley WS, Mustafa RA, Fiander M, et al. Educational games for health professionals. Cochrane Database of Systematic Reviews. 2013;(1): CD006411

[36] Gentile DA, Anderson C. Video games. Encyclopedia of Human Development. 2006;**3**:1303-1307

[37] Greitemeyer T, Osswald S. Effects of prosocial video games on prosocial behavior. Journal of Personality and Social Psychology. 2010;**98**(2):211-221

[38] Thompson D, Baranowskia T, Cullen K, Watson K, Liu Y, Canada A, et al. Food, fun, and fitness internet program for girls: Pilot evaluation of an e-health youth obesity prevention program examining predictors of obesity. Preventive Medicine. 2008; **47**(5):494-497

[39] Buday R, Thompson D, Baranowski T, Lyons EJ. Developing games for health behavior change: Getting started. Games for Health Journal. 2013;**2**(4):83-190

[40] Teed R. Game-based learning. Science Education Resource Center of Carlet Collection. 2012;**15**. Available from: https://serc.carleton.edu/introgeo/games/index.html

[41] Ketelhut DJ. The impact of student self-efficacy on scientific inquiry skills: An exploratory investigation in River City, a multi-user virtual environment. Journal of science education and technology. 1 February 2007;**16**(1): 99-111

[42] Delima R, Arianti NKPB. Identification of user needs for educational game applications for children 4 to 6 years old (in Indonesian). J Tek Inform dan Sist Inf. 2015

[43] James SR, Ashwill J. Nursing Care of Children: Principles and Practice. 3rd ed. Canada: Saunders Elsevie; 2007

[44] Nisa DA, Indrayana. Designing of Board Games as Learning Media for Traffic Signs for Kindergarten Children Aged 5–6 years Old (in Indonesian); 2012

Section 6

Acute Diarrhea and Epilepsy

Chapter 6

Acute Diarrhea as a Manifestation of Abdominal Epilepsy

Tomohiko Murai and Masako Kinoshita

Abstract

Medical doctors are very frequently confronted with gastrointestinal complaints in daily clinical practice. Most of them are ascribed to gastrointestinal disease in general. There exist, however, cases who complain with abdominal signs and symptoms whose causes are unable to be found, in spite of various examinations related to the abdomen. Epilepsy is a chronic disorder of the central nervous system manifesting with recurrent unprovoked seizures. Abnormal abdominal sensation often heralds the onset of epileptic seizures. Among them, there is a rare syndrome called abdominal epilepsy in which episodic gastrointestinal complaints like abdominal pain, abdominal discomfort, nausea, vomit, and diarrhea are the primary or the sole manifestation of epileptic seizures. It is important for clinicians to know that abdominal epilepsy is one of the differential diagnoses of acute gastrointestinal signs and that these symptoms can be treated with antiepileptic medications. Here we review abdominal epilepsy as one of the causes in acute diarrhea.

Keywords: acute diarrhea, recurrent diarrhea, semiology, epileptic seizures

1. Introduction

We clinicians often have to deal with gastrointestinal complaints in daily medical practice. Most of the abnormal abdominal signs and symptoms are ascribed to gastrointestinal disease in general. Meanwhile, the autonomic nervous system is a part of the central nervous system (CNS) and innervates all organs of the body including the gastrointestinal system (**Figure 1**). Autonomic dysfunction manifests with gastrointestinal symptoms like constipation, diarrhea, and oropharyngeal dysphagia. Neurodegenerative disorders as multiple systemic atrophy, allied parkinsonian disorders, and pure autonomic failure can show autonomic manifestations including gastrointestinal signs. Diabetes mellitus and alcoholic enteropathy also cause neurogenic diarrhea along with anxiety neurosis [1]. Their symptoms are usually chronic.

There are, however, rare cases with gastrointestinal manifestations whose causes cannot be found, though various examinations related to the abdomen are performed. Their symptoms are acute and recurrent episodically. Epileptic seizures are a “transient occurrence of signs and/or symptoms due to abnormal excessive or synchronous neuronal activity in the brain” [2]. Epileptic seizures have to be distinguished from nonepileptic seizures and acute provoked seizures that occurs in the context of an acute brain damage or systemic disorder, such as, but not limited to, stroke, head trauma, a toxic or metabolic insult, or an intracranial infection [3].

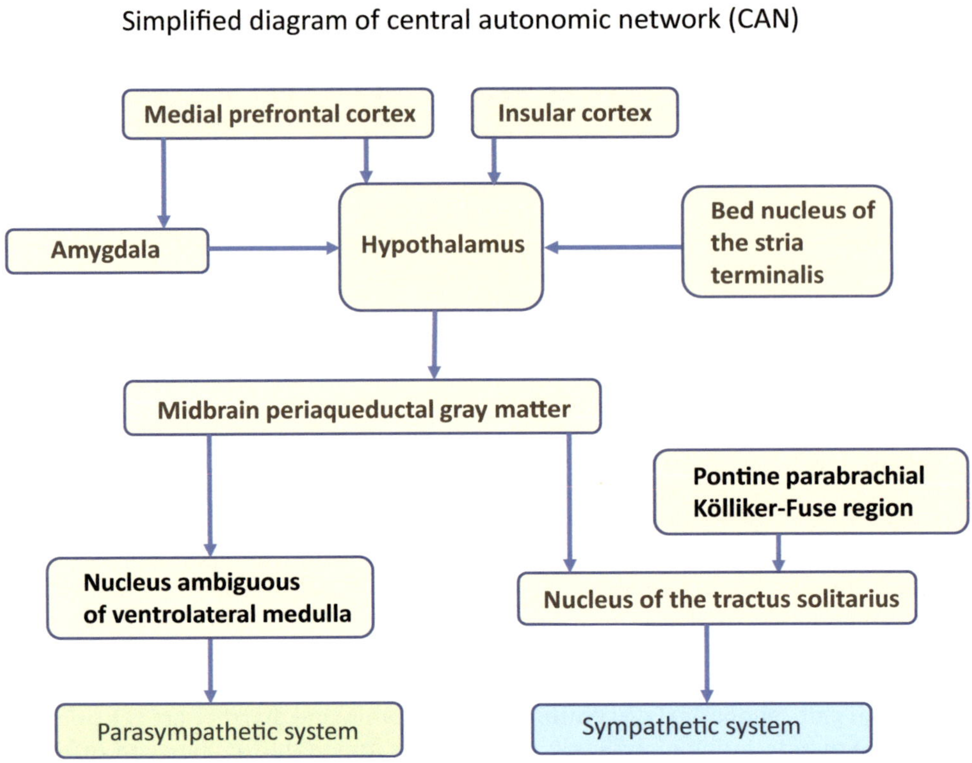

Figure 1.
Simplified diagram of central autonomic network (CAN).

In the widely accepted operational definition of epilepsy, it requires that an individual has at least two provoked seizures on separate days, generally 24 hours apart. There are various seizure types in accord with the cortical function of the epileptic foci and propagated areas in epilepsy. Abnormal abdominal sensation often heralds the onset of epileptic seizures. Among them, there is a rare syndrome called abdominal epilepsy in which episodic gastrointestinal complaints like abdominal pain, abdominal discomfort, nausea, vomit, and diarrhea are the primary or the sole manifestation of epileptic seizures. It is important for clinicians to know that abdominal epilepsy is one of the differential diagnoses of gastrointestinal signs, especially when they are acute onset and recurrent, and that it is treatable with antiepileptic medications.

Here we review abdominal epilepsy as one of the causes in acute diarrhea.

2. Definition

Abdominal epilepsy is characterized by paroxysmal gastrointestinal signs and symptoms resulting from epileptic activity of the neurons in the brain. Epileptic seizures of several patients with abdominal epilepsy are accompanied with impairment of the CNS like loss of consciousness and headache. There is no authorized diagnosis criterion for abdominal epilepsy at present. Zinkin and Peppercorn propose the following criteria for diagnosis of abdominal epilepsy. That is to say, (1) paroxysmal gastrointestinal manifestations of undetermined origin after thorough evaluation including laboratory, radiographic, and endoscopy testing, (2) symptoms originated from the CNS, (3) an abnormal electroencephalogram (EEG) findings relatively specific for epileptic seizures, and (4) a sustained improvement of symptoms by antiepileptic medication [4].

Though many authors cite this criterion in their case reports published hitherto, there are several points at issue in this definition as follows. The gastrointestinal symptoms as acute symptomatic seizures should be ruled out; i.e., unprovoked chronic recurrence or more than 60% probability to recur is needed to diagnose epilepsy [5]. It is difficult to certify the diagnosis by EEG findings (difficulty to record in ictal state, difficulty to record EEG activities via scalp electrodes in cases with epileptogenic foci on mesial temporal area or insular cortex especially in small areas, and low rate of detecting the epileptogenic discharge on patient with epilepsy in general). In case of refractory epilepsy, symptoms could not be improved by antiepileptic drug. Therefore new definition is expected to capture the real entity of this disease.

3. Epidemiology

Hitherto, publications concerning abdominal epilepsy are quite limited in number. Accurate prevalence rate of abdominal epilepsy has not been evaluated. There are 36 cases reported in literature, in the review of abdominal epilepsy by Zinkin and Peppercorn [4]. We found other 15 cases of abdominal epilepsy in

author	published year	Age	Gender	gastrointestinal symptoms	CNS symptoms	MRI/CT	SPECT	EEG	laterality on EEG	abnormal location on EEG	treatment
Scotinotis	2000	66	M	nausea	none	unremarkable	NA	sharp wave	right	temporal	CBZ
Topno	2005	38	F	abdominal pain	LOC, post-ictal amnesia	unremarkable	NA	sharp wave	right	fronto-temporal	PHE
Shihabuddin	2007	72	F	abdominal pain, nausea	none	NA	NA	ictal discharge	right	temporal	LTG
Dutta	2007	50	M	abdominal discomfort, vomit	NA	unremarkable	NA	dysrhythmia in the form slowing	left	temporal	OXC
		52	F	abdominal discomfort, vomit	headache, drowsiness	unremarkable	NA	focal discharge with generalization	right	frontal	OXC
Sekimoto	2007	32	M	nausea, vomit	palpitation	unremarkable	NA	low voltage spikes	bilateral	occipital, parietal	CBZ
		23	F	nausea, vomit	vaguely unpleasant feeling	unremarkable	NA	low voltage spikes	bilateral	occipital, parietal	CBZ
Tiamkao	2011	20	F	abdominal pain, nausea	GTCS	NA	NA	sharp wave	NA	NA	PHE, DIA
		46	M	epigastric pain, vomit	none	NA	NA	spike	NA	NA	PHE
		21	F	abdominal discomfort, vomit	none	NA	NA	spike	NA	NA	PHE
Murai	2014	63	F	abdominal discomfort, diarrhea	LOC, palpitation	unremarkable	decreased blood flow in the left frontal and temporal	sharp transients, delta waves	left	anterior-mid temporal	CBZ
Harshe	2016	45	F	abdominal pain, vomit	none	NA	NA	spike and slow wave complexes	bilateral	NA	VPA
Hayashida	2016	71	F	nausea, vomit	headache	unremarkable	perfusion defects in the frontotemporo parietal	sharp wave	left	temporal	LEV, CZP
Mpondo	2016	38	M	abdominal pain	none	NA	NA	spikes	bilateral	temporal	CBZ
Al-Hail	2018	26	F	abdonminal pain	none	left mesial temporal sclerosis	NA	sharp wave	left	anterior temporal	LTG

Abbreviations: LOC, loss of consciousness; GTCS, generalized tonic-clonic seizure; NA, not available; CBZ, carbamazepine; PHE, phenytoin; LTG, lamotorigine; OXC, oxcarbazepine; DIA, diazepam; VPA, sodium valporate; CZP, clonazepam

Table 1.
Summary of case reports by literature.

English literature after Zinkin's review paper [6–16]. In the reported cases, there is no racial specificity nor regional specificity. The number of patients with abdominal epilepsy could be more than reported cases because the entity of abdominal epilepsy has still not been recognized and because nonmotor seizure manifestations are often underdiagnosed. **Table 1** shows the patient profile of 15 case reports that was published after his review. Elderly patients of more than 60 years old are only 1 case (2%) out of his 36 cases and 4 cases (26%) out of 15 cases. Recently there is increasing evidence that elderly with dementia have greater risk of epilepsy. Hayashida et al. reported that the cumulative incidence of at least one unprovoked seizure in individuals with Alzheimer's disease is in the range of 10–20% [14]. From now on, the number of abdominal epilepsy could be increased along with the increase of elderly patients with epilepsy.

4. Clinical features

Abdominal epilepsy is quite uncommon. Zinkin and Peppercorn found only 36 reported cases in the English literature since Douglas and White laid the groundwork in the reporting of cases of abdominal epilepsy in 1971, and they reviewed 36 patients with abdominal epilepsy in the past 34 years [4]. After their report, we found other 15 adult cases in English literature (**Table 1**). Age of patients varies a great deal from 1 to 71 years, and female is 57% (29/51), without any significant predisposition. Gastrointestinal manifestations of epilepsy include abdominal pain in 76% (39/51), nausea and/or vomit in 43% (22/51), and diarrhea in 6% (3/51); in abdominal epilepsy, rate of occurrence of diarrhea is quite rare as a gastrointestinal symptom. All three patients with diarrhea had the abnormal findings on EEG in temporal area. Antiepileptic drugs were prescribed (phenobarbital, valproic acid, and carbamazepine). The outcome was complete resolution or well-controlled.

5. Examination

General physical examination is unremarkable. The examination directly related with gastrointestinal signs and symptoms, for example, abdominal computed tomography (CT) scan, abdominal ultrasound, and gastrointestinal endoscopy, is normal. Blood tests and cerebrospinal fluid examination are usually normal.

Neuroimaging like magnetic resonance (MR) imaging and/or CT scan or single-photon emission computed tomography (SPECT) sometimes shows local lesion, especially in temporal areas. Two cases have no remarkable MR imaging and/or CT but abnormal findings in temporal lobe or areas including temporal lobe on brain SPECT (one, decreased blood flow in the left frontal and temporal; the other, perfusion defects in the frontotemporal-parietal area) [12, 14]. There is one patient who has abnormal lesion in temporal lobe on MR imaging (left mesial temporal sclerosis) [16]. No specific finding is relevant to diagnosis of abdominal epilepsy.

As is the case with any type of epilepsy, EEG is one of the most important examinations for abdominal epilepsy. EEG is a record of the electrical potentials generated in neurons from electrodes attached to the human scalp. One estimate is that approximately 6 cm^2 of cortical surface must be synchronously activated in order for there to be a potential recorded at the surface [17]. Abnormal EEG activity can be classified into two types: epileptiform and non-epileptiform. The two most important types of abnormal activity are slowing and epileptiform activity. Slow waves indicate disordered function of the neuron, whereas epileptiform activities indicate abnormal synchronous activity [17]. EEG is of diagnostic power when significant epileptiform discharges are detected. Spikes and sharp waves are epileptiform discharges that reflect the paroxysmal depolarization shifts in the epileptic neurons. They are basically surface negative but in rare occasions surface positive. Patients with epilepsy has abnormal EEG findings even though they are in interictal state. Interictal epileptic discharge like spikes and sharp waves is recognized on EEG of abdominal epilepsy patients; however, less specific EEG changes can be a clue for diagnosis.

In patients with epilepsy, generally speaking, the initial EEG examination shows interictal epileptiform discharges in only about 50%; therefore, normal EEG does not exclude the presence of epileptic disorder. It is hard to capture the abnormal signals in case of deeper lesion and/or small foci in the brain. As for enhancement of sensitivity, the detection rate is increased by performing repeated EEG at different times or by physiological activation procedures like hyperventilation, sleep recording, and photic stimulation. Long-term video EEG monitoring is one of the useful tools for diagnosis of epilepsy. Video EEG monitoring is an EEG record with video recording continuously for several days including sleep in the night and performed for direct correlation of clinical symptoms with EEG findings. When the gastrointestinal signs and symptoms occur and abnormal EEG findings (epileptiform discharge) are recognized at the same time, the diagnosis of epilepsy is determined. In most of the reports in the past, abnormal findings on EEG are interictal, but only one case report has ictal EEG recording showing left anterior temporal onset [16].

6. Pathophysiology

Seizure semiology of abdominal epilepsy is usually categorized as partial seizures (simple partial seizures with preserved consciousness, complex partial seizures with impaired consciousness, and secondarily generalized seizures with loss of consciousness and generalized convulsion) [4]. Based on the operational classification of seizure types by the International League Against Epilepsy (ILAE) (2017), epileptic seizures with onset of autonomic features are classified into autonomic (onset) seizures. According to the "ILAE classification of the epilepsies: Position paper of the ILAE Commission for Classification and Terminology," [18] abdominal epilepsy is categorized as a focal epilepsy, whatever the etiology may be.

In history, many cases have been described, and many terms have been used for paroxysmal autonomic symptoms including gastrointestinal ones classified as epilepsy from the times of Armand Trousseau [19]. Moore used the term abdominal epilepsy for the first time for patients with abdominal pain or abdominal pain with nausea and vomit caused by epileptic seizures [20]. Because sensory symptoms are related to loss of consciousness or any other impairment of central nervous system, the sensory symptoms are regarded as an aura [21].

The mechanism that abdominal epilepsy occurs is still unclear, but several studies indicate that temporal lobe structures including the amygdala and hippocampus, insular cortex, and limbic systems could be related with inducing abdominal sign and symptoms known as abdominal epilepsy [4]. Ictal autonomic changes are probably due to direct excitation or inhibition of neocortex and limbic systems involved in seizure onset and their propagation to structures that constitute the central autonomic network (**Figure 1**) [21]. The brain controls widespread autonomic responses through the central autonomic network ranging from the cerebral hemisphere to the brain stem. The insular and medial prefrontal cortices, the hippocampus, and the amygdala are the major inputs to transmit cortical activity to the central nervous network. Certain autonomic symptoms and signs (vomiting, nausea, and alterations in heart rate and respiration, flushing, sweating, piloerection, pupil dilatation) indicate specific localization and lateralization of the seizure-onset zone [21–24].

7. Diagnosis

Gastrointestinal disease should be ruled out at first. The detail of history as recurrent paroxysmal episodes of gastrointestinal symptoms is needed for the diagnosis of abdominal epilepsy. The duration of symptoms is usually within a few minutes. It is important to distinguish abdominal epilepsy itself from abdominal auras preceding to other major seizure manifestations of temporal or parieto-occipital epilepsies [23].

On the contrary, information of subjective findings related to epileptic auras should be carefully obtained. Especially, epigastric rising sensation, déjà vu, jamais vu, olfactory sensation, and sudden emergence of certain memory are related to temporal lobe epilepsy. When gastrointestinal symptoms and signs are the sole seizure manifestation, nonepileptic disease could be included in the differential diagnosis since gastrointestinal signs may often be wrongly diagnosed. Ictal autonomic symptoms are most often associated with epileptiform discharges in limbic portions of the temporal and frontal lobes on EEG [25].

8. Treatment

There has been no controlled trial that provides evidence-based medication on treatment of abdominal epilepsy so far. Treatment is the same as other types of epilepsy, and antiepileptic drug is usually used. Epileptic seizures of abdominal epilepsy are recognized as one of the partial seizures; therefore, carbamazepine or phenytoin is selected as the first line in medication. If the first drug is not effective enough, the certain drug would be increased to the maximum tolerable dose, or other types of medication can be added on, based on the patient's response.

9. Prognosis

The prognosis of abdominal epilepsy is generally good. In most patients, antiepileptic drug is effective, and only antiepileptic medication brings relief in gastrointestinal symptoms. In cases who are drug-resistant to single medication, polytherapy is needed by using a couple of antiepileptic drugs in combination. Other kinds of autonomic signs and symptoms, and seizure manifestations other than autonomic features, might also reflect a reaction to the occurrence of epileptic seizures [23]. Therefore, it is necessary to check subjective/objective findings by thorough medical history taking and to schedule follow-up examinations including EEG evaluation.

10. Conclusions

Patients with focal epilepsy often exhibit a variety of autonomic symptoms including abdominal sensations as auras (simple partial seizures, or focal seizures with retained awareness). When gastrointestinal complaints, usually abdominal pain and nausea, are the most prominent manifestation of epileptic seizures, they are called as abdominal epilepsy. Abdominal epilepsy should be suspected as one of the possible diagnoses in patients with diarrhea and other autonomic symptoms, even though they do not exhibit convulsions or other typical motor manifestations. Unless a careful and detailed history taking reveals the subjective and objective findings by patients and witnesses, a possible diagnosis of epilepsy and a therapeutic trial of antiepileptic therapy are never considered. Detection of significant epileptiform discharges in EEG is the cardinal method for diagnosis; however, normal EEG does not exclude the possibility of epileptic disorders because only half of patients with clinical diagnosis of epileptic seizures or epilepsy show overt abnormality. Subtle EEG findings, especially reproducible ones whose distribution is in concordance with clinical manifestations, should not be neglected. Acute diarrhea as one of the manifestations of focal epilepsy, especially temporal lobe epilepsy, is quite uncommon, but it is important to recognize the clinical entity.

Acknowledgements

No funding for this paper.

Conflict of interest

The authors have no conflict of interests to disclose.

Author details

Tomohiko Murai[1] and Masako Kinoshita[2]*

1 Department of Neurology, Kyoto City Hospital, Kyoto, Japan

2 Department of Neurology, Utano National Hospital, National Hospital Organization, Kyoto, Japan

*Address all correspondence to: machak@kuhp.kyoto-u.ac.jp

References

[1] Mathias CJ, Freeman R. Autonomic dysfunction. In: Neurological Disorders: Course and Treatment. 2nd ed. Cambridge: Academic Press; 2003

[2] Fisher RS, Boas W, et al. Epileptic seizures and epilepsy: Definition proposed by the International League against Epilepsy (ILAE) and the International Bureau for Epilepsy (IBE). Epilepsia. 2005;**46**:470. DOI: 10.1111/j.0013-9580.2005.66104.x

[3] Guideline for epidemiologic studies on epilepsy. Commission on Epidemiology and Prognosis, International League Against Epilepsy. Epilepsia. 1993;**34**:592-596

[4] Zinkin NT, Peppercorn MA. Abdominal epilepsy. Best Practice & Research Clinical Gastroenterology. 2005;**19**:263-274. DOI: 10.1016/j.bpg.2004.10.001

[5] Fisher RS, Acevedo C, et al. ILAE official report: A practical clinical definition of epilepsy. Epilepsia. 2014;**55**:475-482. DOI: 10.1111/epi.12550

[6] Scotiniotis I, Stecker M, et al. Recurrent nausea as part of the spectrum of abdominal epilepsy. Digestive Diseases and Sciences. 2000;**45**:1238-1240

[7] Topno N, Gopasetty MS, et al. Abdominal epilepsy and foreign body in the abdominal dilemma in diagnosis of abdominal pain. Yonsei Medical Journal. 2005;**46**:870-873. DOI: 10.3349/ymj.2005.46.6.870

[8] Shihabuddin BS, Harik SI. Episodic nausea and abdominal sensations as sole manifestations of simple partial seizures. Neurosciences. 2007;**12**:327-329

[9] Dutta SR, Hazarika I, Chakravarty BP. Abdominal epilepsy, an uncommon cause of recurrent abdominal pain: A brief report. Gut. 2007;**56**:439-441. DOI: 10.1136/gut.2006.094250

[10] Sekimoto M, kato M, et al. Ictal nausea with vomiting as the major symptom of simple partial seizures: Electroencephalographic and magnetoencephalographic analysis. Epilepsy and Behavior. 2007;**11**:582-587. DOI: 10.1016/j.yebeh.2007.08.023

[11] Tiamkao S, Pratipanawatr T, et al. Abdominal epilepsy: An uncommon of non-convulsive status epilepticus. Journal of the Medical Association of Thailand. 2011;**94**:998-1001

[12] Murai T, Tohyama T, Kinoshita M. Recurrent diarrhea as a manifestation of temporal lobe epilepsy. Epilepsy and Behavior Case Reports. 2014;**2**:57-59. DOI: 10.1016/j.ebcr.2014.03.007

[13] Harshe DG, Harshe SD, et al. Abdominal epilepsy in an adult: A diagnosis often missed. Journal of Clinical and Diagnostic Research. 2016;**10**:VD01-VD02. DOI: 10.7860/JCDR/2016/19873.8600

[14] Hayashida A, Tomizawa Y, et al. Abdominal epilepsy associated with Alzheimer's disease. Journal of the American Geriatrics Society. 2016;**64**(5):1146-1147. DOI: 10.1111/jgs.14125

[15] Mpondo BC, Mwasada G, et al. Abdominal epilepsy, an uncommon cause of chronic and recurrent abdominal pain: A case report. Clinical Case Reports. 2016;**4**:1117-1119. DOI: 10.1002.ccr3.711

[16] Al-Hail H, Wilkins SS, et al. Temporal epilepsy causing recurrent abdominal pain in adults. World Journal of Neuroscience. 2018;**8**:270-276. DOI: 10.4236/wjns.2018.82021

[17] Misulis KE. Atlas of EEG, Seizure Semiology, and Management. 2nd ed.

Oxford: Oxford University Press; 2014. pp. 26-29. DOI: 10.1093/med/97801999985906.001.0001

[18] Fisher RS, Cross JH, et al. Operational classification of seizure types by the International League Against Epilepsy: Position Paper of the ILAE Commission for Classification and Terminology. Epilepsia. 2017;**58**: 522-530. DOI: 10.1111/epi.13670

[19] Moseley B, Bateman L, et al. Autonomic epileptic seizures, autonomic effects of seizures and SUDEP. Epilepsy and Behavior. 2013;**26**: 375-385. DOI: 10.1016/j.2012.08.020

[20] Moore MT. Abdominal epilepsy. The Review of Gastroenterology. 1948; **15**:381-395

[21] Peppercorn MA, Herzog AG. The spectrum of abdominal epilepsy in adults. The American Journal of Gastroenterology. 1989;**84**:1294-1296

[22] Tufenkjian K, Luders HO. Seizure semiology: Its value and limitations in localizing the epileptogenic zone. Journal of Clinical Neurology. 2012;**8**: 243-250. DOI: 10.3988/jcn.2012.8.4.243

[23] Foldvary-Schaefer N, Unnwongse K. Localizing and lateralizing features of auras and seizures. Epilepsy and Behavior. 2011;**20**:160-166. DOI: 10.1016/j.yebeh.2010.08.034

[24] Freeman R, Schachter SC. Autonomic epilepsy. Seminars in Neurology. 1995;**15**:158-166. DOI: 10.1055/s-2008-1041019

[25] Engel JJR. Seizures and Epilepsy. Oxford: Oxford University Press; 2013. p. 210. DOI: 10.1093/med/9780195328547.001.0001